HEALTH AND WORK

Also by Lesley Doyal

What Makes Women Sick: Gender and the Political Economy of Health

HEALTH AND WORK

CRITICAL PERSPECTIVES

edited by

Norma Daykin and Lesley Doyal

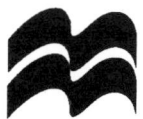

First published in Great Britain 1999 by
MACMILLAN PRESS LTD
Houndmills, Basingstoke, Hampshire RG21 6XS and London
Companies and representatives throughout the world

A catalogue record for this book is available from the British Library.

ISBN 0–333–69190–3 hardcover
ISBN 0–333–69191–1 paperback

First published in the United States of America 1999 by
ST. MARTIN'S PRESS, INC.,
Scholarly and Reference Division,
175 Fifth Avenue, New York, N.Y. 10010

ISBN 0–312–22342–0

Library of Congress Cataloging-in-Publication Data
Health and work : critical perspectives / edited by Norma Daykin and
Lesley Doyal.
p.   cm.
Includes bibliographical references and index.
ISBN 0–312–22342–0 (cloth)
1. Industrial hygiene.   I. Daykin, Norma.   II. Doyal, Lesley.
RC967.H425   1999
616.9'803—dc21   99–19219
                                                              CIP

This book is printed on paper suitable for recycling and made from fully managed and
sustained forest sources.

10   9   8   7   6   5   4   3   2   1
08   07   06   05   04   03   02   01   00   99

Printed in Hong Kong

CONTENTS

NOTES ON CONTRIBUTORS

Joyce E. Canaan is Senior Lecturer in the Sociology Department at the University of Central England. She has published numerous chapters in the area of the ethnography of education and has recently co-edited (with Debbie Epstein) *A Question of Discipline: Pedagogy and Power in the Teaching of Cultural Studies* (Westview: Boulder, Colorado and Oxford, UK, 1997). She has also recently completed a study with Baljit Kaur Basatia and Surinder Kaur of the AEKTA Project in Birmingham, funded by the Barrol-Cadbury Foundation, entitled *The Double Burden Intensified: Asian Women Homeworkers' Perceptions of their Pay and Conditions* (1999).

Nick J. Fox is Senior Lecturer in sociology in the School of Health and Related Research (ScHARR) at the University of Sheffield. He is the author of *The Social Meaning of Surgery* (Open University Press, 1992) and *Postmodernism, Sociology and Health* (Open University Press, 1993). He has written extensively on postmodern social theory as applied to health and care and is currently completing a new book in this field entitled *Beyond Health: Blueprint for a Postmodern Embodiment* (Free Association Books, 1999).

Christer Hogstedt is Professor of Occupational Health at the Swedish National Institute for Working Life and directs NIWL's multi-disciplinary Department for Work and Health. He is also senior physician at the Karolinska Hospital and at the Labour Inspectorate, both in Stockholm. He has served as expert advisor on environmental health to the Swedish Government's Ministry of Health and Social Welfare and as president of the Swedish Association for Occupational Health and Safety in Developing Countries. He has also served as consultant to several international bodies including the World Health Organisation and the International Commission on Occupational Health. He has edited 14 books (five international) and published over 200 scientific articles as well as numerous papers and contributions at international conferences.

Asa C. Laurell is Professor of Social Medicine at the Autonomous Metropolitan University in Mexico City. Her professional training is in medicine and she has an MPH and a PhD in Sociology. She has published extensively on work process and health as well as health policy and social security reform. Her publications include the books *La Salud en la Fabrica* (Health in the Factory) and *La Reforma contra la Salud y la Seguridad Social* (The Reform against Health and Social Security). She has also served as a consultant to trade unions and to the Commissions of Health and Social Security of the Mexican Congress.

Liz Lloyd is a Lecturer in Community Care in the School for Policy Studies at the University of Bristol. She is the author of a number of journal articles and papers on health and social care services for elderly people. Her current research is on community care for elderly people through the process of dying.

Dr Rene Loewenson is a Zimbabwean epidemiologist. She has worked as a Senior Lecturer in the Department of Community Medicine at the University of Zimbabwe Medical School; as Head of the Zimbabwe Congress of Trade Unions Health and Social Welfare Department and as Technical Co-ordinator for the Organisation of African Trade Union Unity, Health, Safety and Environment Programme. She is currently Director of the Training and Research Support Centre in Zimbabwe. She has researched and published on issues related to health, economic policy and employment from both an occupational health and public health perspective.

Karen Messing is a Professor of Biology at the University of Quebec at Montreal and a researcher at CINBIOSE (the Centre for the Study of Biological Interactions in Environmental Health). She has published many articles on various aspects of occupational health in jobs occupied by women, and carried out research in partnership with Quebec unions, her most recent book being *One Eyed Science: Occupational Health and Women Workers*, published by Temple University Press in 1998.

Theo Nichols is Professor of Sociology at the University of Bristol and Editor of the journal *Work, Employment and Society*. He has written widely in the area of economic sociology. His recent publications include *Work and Occupation in Modern Turkey* (edited with Erol Kahveci and Nadir Sugur, 1996) and *The Sociology of Industrial Injury* (1997).

Sarah Payne lectures in health policy at the School for Policy Studies, University of Bristol. Her research interests include gender and mental health issues in the delivery of mental health services, and inequalities in health and deprivation, particularly in relation to women's experience of poverty and the experience of deprivation in rural areas.

Simon Pickvance has worked as an Occupational Health Advisor in the primary care system in Sheffield since 1980. He is also a Senior Research Fellow at the Centre for Environmental and Occupational Health Policy at De Montfort University and co-editor of the *Workers' Health International Newsletter*. Recent publications include contributions to the International Labour Organisation *Encyclopedia of Occupational Health and Safety* and a handbook on Occupational Health and Safety for Steelworkers.

Ruth Pinder is Associate Research Fellow at the Centre for the Study of Health, Brunel University, and Research Fellow at Queen Mary Westfield College, University of London. She has published widely in the field of chronic illness and disability, including *The Management of Chronic Illness: Patients' and Doctors' Perspectives on Parkinson's Disease*. She is also an Education Consultant and runs workshops on disability and gender for health care professionals within the British Postgraduate Medical Federation.

Annette Scambler has taught sociology and women's studies for the Open University for 15 years. She has honorary lectureships at University College London and at Imperial College, and she was a Visiting Professor in the Department of Sociology at Emory University, Atlanta, USA, in 1998. She has researched women's health issues, her publications including: (as co-author) *Menstrual Disorders* (Routledge, 1993) and (as co-editor) *Rethinking Prostitution: Purchasing Sex in the 1990s* (Routledge, 1997).

Graham Scambler is Reader in Sociology and Director of the Unit of Medical Sociology at University College London. He was a Visiting Professor in the Department of Sociology at Emory University, Atlanta, USA, in 1998. His interests include social theory, health inequalities, chronic and stigmatizing illness, and the sex industry. Recent publications include: (as editor) *Sociology as Applied to Medicine* (4th edn, Saunders, 1997); (as co-editor) *Rethinking Prostitution: Purchasing Sex* *in the 1990s* (Routledge, 1997); and (as co-editor) *Modernity, Medicine and Health: Medical Sociology Towards 2000* (Routledge, 1998).

Andrew Watterson is Professor of Occupational and Environmental Health and Director of the Centre for Occupational and Environmental Health at De Montfort University, Leicester, where he is also Head of the Department of Health and Continuing Professional Studies. He is a registered safety practitioner, his research interests lying in inter-disciplinary approaches to occupational and environmental health, especially lay and worker epidemiology and toxicology. He has published widely in this field, including the second edition of *The Role of the Health and Safety Manager* (with Les Wright) in 1998.

Tamsin Wilton is Reader in the Sociology of Sex and Sexualities in the School of Health Sciences at the University of the West of England. Her publications include *En/Gendering AIDS: Deconstructing Sex, Text and Epidemic*; *Finger Licking Good: The Ins and Outs of Lesbian Sex*; and (edited with Lesley Doyal and Jennie Naidoo) *AIDS: Setting a Feminist Agenda*. Her textbook on sexuality for health and social care professionals will be published by the Open University Press in 1999.

PREFACE

The impetus for this book came from several sources. At one level we were both aware of a number of theoretical and methodological assumptions that have impeded the study of health and work. We also recognised the increasing need for interdisciplinary collaboration in order to align the separate foci of the various contributing disciplines. While specialist literature addresses technical problems within the workplace, it often overloks the social dimensions of risk. Similarly, psychologists have studied the impact of work stress on individuals but have paid less attention to the broader social processes involved in the construction of occupational health and disease. As far as sociology is concerned, research on labour markets and processes is well established but often seems to be founded on the assumption that it is the economic consequences of work that matter. While medical sociologists have examined the socioeconomic determinants of health, and highlighted employment status as a marker of broad social divisions, they have paid relatively little attention to the health effects of work itself.

These problems are compounded by those arising from reliance on limited and outmoded definitions of 'work'. Feminist critiques of this focus on paid employment in the productive sphere are now familiar but they are yet to enter mainstream research and practice in the field of occupational health. Finally, biological reductionism and technological determinism have often rendered occupational health research and practice unable to respond to the increasingly complex, chronic and multicausal nature of work-related ill health.

The problems of serial invisibility are responsible for various forms of epidemiological bias in occupational health research that are addressed in this book. The book aims to introduce interdisciplinary and global perspectives to the study of work and risk in order to inform both theory and practice. It is intended for students of social and health sciences as well as researchers, practitioners and policy makers in all the fields relating to health and work.

It is perhaps ironic that this project arose out of experiences very similar to some of those described in the pages that follow; the lack of awareness of many health professionals about occupational health issues; the inadequacy or non-existence of workplace occupational health services; the difficulty of reconciling 'lay' and 'expert' views amd the harmfulness of some well meaning but non-evidence-based clinical interventions. One of us (Norma Daykin) had the misfortune to experience these at first hand, an experience which led her to initiate the discussions between us which led to the idea for the book.

The book also testifies to the possibility of rehabilitation, underpinned in this case by the support and collaboration of colleagues, the availability of appropriate technical support, the reflexivity and skill of some (orthodox and complementary) health practitioners and, not least, the encouragement of students and friends. Special thanks are due to Nick Fox and Tamsin Wilton whose enthusiasm and support helped to relaunch the idea at a critical time and to Lorraine ayensu who never wavered in her belief and encouragement. We are also grateful to colleagues who helped in practical ways, in particular Jenny Dafforn and Julie Packer at the University of the West, both of whom gave invaluable secretarial support. Not least, thanks are due to the staff at Macmillan, in particular Houri Alavi whose efficiency and interest in the project helped sustain it until completion.

ACKNOWLEDGEMENTS

The authors and publishers wish to thank the following for permission to use copyright material:

Frank Cass Publishers for Figure 5.9 from *Middle Eastern Studies*, 31(2).

HMSO for Figure 11.1 from *A Guide to Risk Management for Environmental Protection*, 1995, Crown Copyright.

London Hazard Centre for Table 6.6 from *The Asbestos Hazards Handbook*, 1995.

Rory O'Neill for Table 6.3 from *Asthma at Work*, 1995, Hazard Publications.

WHO European Centre for Environment and Health for Tables 6.2 and 6.4 from *Concern for Europe's Tomorrow* and *Health and the Environment in the WHO European Region*. Stuttgart, Wissenschaftliche Verlagsgesellschaft, 1995.

Every effort has been made to trace all the copyright holders, but if any have been inadvertently overlooked the publishers will be pleased to make the necessary arrangement at the first opportunity.

INTRODUCTION: CRITICAL PERSPECTIVES ON HEALTH AND WORK

Norma Daykin

Traditional understandings of the relationship between health and work have been called into question in what has variously been termed late modern, high modern and postmodern society. Conventional models, developed in the context of western industrial societies, are based on notions of work that fail to account for the experience of growing numbers of individuals. They also draw on ideas about the nature of science that have been challenged from a number of perspectives. Finally, they assume modes of political organisation which can no longer be taken for granted in societies where risks are often global and yet individuals' experience of work may be more and more fragmented.

These shifts represent significant challenges to health researchers, policy makers and activists. They are addressed in differing ways by the contributors to this book who are drawn from a wide range of backgrounds including the academic disciplines of social and human science and occupational health practice and activism. Given this diversity, it is neither possible nor desirable to offer a unified theory or a single set of prescriptions for addressing problems of health and work. Rather, a deliberately eclectic approach is taken here, drawing on the strengths of this wide range of perspectives. The general aim of the book is to question and extend the basis of knowledge and practice around health and work in response to changing concepts and patterns of risk that increasingly limit the value of traditional approaches.

Understanding work and risk

Traditional understandings of the relationship between health and work have drawn upon relatively narrow models of work. For example, they have focused on paid employment in the productive sector to the exclusion of many other arenas of labour, particularly those occupied by women (Tancred, 1995). There are many other activities which could be defined as work but these are usually ignored both in research and policies for health and safety in employment. Such activities may, for example, mirror forms of paid employment but be unpaid, such as caring for dependants or performing domestic work within the household (Doyal, 1995 and this volume; Lloyd, this volume; Payne, this volume). They may involve unrecognised physical and psychological risks similar to those of paid employment, as well as specific risks, such as isolation, arising from the social setting in which they are carried out. Conventional research and provision also neglects forms of work which lie outside the formal, regulated sector even if these involve the exchange of money. For example, sex work is often overlooked as a form of labour with attendant risks and hazards (Whittaker and Hart, 1996; see also Scambler and Scambler, this volume and Wilton, this volume).

This debate suggests that notions of work are socially constructed and the same can be said of concepts of health and risk. Social constructionist perspectives draw attention to the ways in which everyday knowledge about reality is created through the interactions and interpretations of individuals, rather than reflecting preexisting 'facts' (Berger and Luckman, 1967; Nettleton, 1995). Hence the meanings attached to health and work (and the actions consequent upon them) are constantly negotiated rather than given. This applies to the labelling of health and illness behaviour within the workplace (Virtanen, 1994) as well as to the attribution of occupational causes to ill health and accidents (Green, 1992). For example, a study of white-collar workers in France demonstrated that the moral evaluation of sick employees by peers and superiors depends not only upon the biological reality of illness but on preexisting attitudes and patterns of power and control (Dodier, 1985). This has profound implications for the wellbeing and rehabilitation of those with both job-related and non-job-related illness and impairments in the workplace (Pinder, 1995 and this volume).

While concepts of 'work', 'health' and 'risk' may be relatively fluid, it is still important to recognise that material conditions affect health too. Attention is now being paid to the ways in which changing patterns of employment are creating new patterns of production and distribution of risks and hazards, presenting opportunities and problems for occupational health researchers, practitioners and activists. A number of global trends have been identified including regional shifts in economic power, sectoral shifts from manufacturing to service industries and technological developments such as those in the chemical and microelectronics industries (Takala, 1995).

The concentration of economic power together with the mobility of capital and resources has led to the globalisation of many occupational hazards. The transfer of traditional and new manufacturing risks to third world countries by multinational corporations attracted by low production costs, weak labour organisation and the lack of regulatory systems is a continuing cause for concern (Elling, 1981; Packard, 1989; Levenstein et al., 1995). For example, as legislation in the USA and Europe has restricted the use of asbestos, the manufacture of asbestos-containing products has shifted to developing countries where regulation is limited (Johanning et al., 1994). This adds to the burden of occupational ill health which is already much greater in these societies than in industrial countries (Levy and Wegman, 1995; Fatusi and Erharbor, 1996). However, much of this illness is hidden by the lack of systematic data collection and the greater levels of general ill health suffered by the working populations of poor countries (Levy and Wegman, 1995; Takala, 1995).

The impact of globalisation is different in different countries and may even benefit some groups of workers. For example, Greenlund and Elling (1995) analysed US data from a national sample to find that workers in companies with a high level of international activity had lower exposure to occupational hazards than their counterparts in local US industries. In other words, foreign investment was inversely related to workplace health and safety problems. This was seen as the consequence of the transfer of hazardous activities and processes to underdeveloped nations and the concentration of health and safety investment in developed countries in response to the demands of organised labour.

These apparent benefits of globalisation for workers in industrialised countries may be offset by some of the costs, however. In these countries, where is often a relatively well developed regulatory framework and infrastructure for addressing problems of health and safety at work, concern has been expressed about the ways in which globalisation undermines the regulatory power of governments (Levenstein et al., 1995; see also Pickvance, this volume). In addition, researchers have explored the ways in which global competition has contributed to the growth of structural unemployment and changes in the labour process, including the intensification of work and the growth of 'flexible' employment (Cameron, 1995). A recent European study noted a common trend towards a decline in 'standard' employment with increased use of part-time working, homeworking, subcontracting and self-employment (Brewster *et al.*, 1997).

The implications of these trends for patterns of occupational illness and disease are now beginning to receive attention from researchers. While there is little room for complacency about 'traditional' occupational disease (see Watterson, this volume), the incidence of established diseases associated with heavy industry, such as asbestosis and pneumoconiosis, is expected to level off in the developed countries with newer problems including occupational asthma, musculoskeletal disorders and stress increasing in relative importance (Artus, 1995). The psychological burdens of work are also perceived to be increasing in societies characterised by the growth of service sector employment (Karasek and Theorell, 1990), and there is a growing interest in issues of mental health in the workplace (Floyd *et al.*, 1994; Williams, 1996; see also Payne, this volume). However, it is difficult to determine the extent to which this reflects a deterioration in the working conditions of articulate groups of white-collar workers (Nichols, 1998). These groups may now be facing stressors, such as lack of job control, which continue to be disproportionately experienced by those in relatively low paid and low status occupations (Nichols, 1998; see also Payne, this volume).

Attention has also been paid to the health implications of changes in work organisation. These can be seen both in terms of problems and opportunities. For example, the intensification of work in some sectors has been linked with increased accident and injury rates (see Canaan, this volume). This is a particular problem for people in non-standard employment, such as the self-employed, and those in the growing number of small firms (Nichols, 1997 and this volume). New forms of labour such as homeworking may bring individual and environmental benefits and costs (Williams, 1996). The benefits cited include reduced exposure to pathogens, increased control over the working environment and reductions in car use. However, it is recognised that homeworking can also lead to increased hours of work in poorly designed workstations, as well as isolation and the loss of relaxation and recovery time.

Insecurity at work has been shown to add to the health burden of individual workers. For example, research on US automobile workers by Heaney *et al.* (1994) found that chronic job insecurity was linked to increased reporting of a range of physical symptoms. A recent UK study (Daykin, 1998) found that uncertainty at work affected individuals' attitudes to occupational health services. Workers were worried that information about their health would be used in decisions about the renewal of contracts as well as promotion and redundancy. As well as these individual effects, the wider social costs of uncertain employment have been explored. Flexibility can transfer risks and costs including pay, training and pensions from the employer to the individual, and ultimately to society, in the form of increased welfare needs among those displaced from standard employment (Brewster *et al.*, 1997). Further, Wilkinson (1996) has suggested that widespread uncertainty may affect population health, undermining progress made in increasing life expectancy in industrialised nations.

The health costs of changing patterns of employment are not shared equally even within industrial societies. Socioeconomic status and health are strongly linked, and recent research in the UK found that men with chronic illness and in manual occupations were more likely than other men to be displaced from the labour market during the 1980s (Bartley and Owen, 1996). Patterns of gender segregation in employment are also strongly linked with the distribution of occupational hazards (Doyal, 1995). An OECD study of ten countries found a consistent and enduring pattern with women concentrated in particular industries and sectors; in lower paid and lower status jobs; and in part-time 'flexible' work (OECD, 1993). A recent study of health and working conditions in the European Union found that women were particularly likely to be involved in precarious or insecure work (Lagerlof, 1997).

Ethnicity is also linked with patterns of insecurity and risk. For example, research in the USA shows that minority ethnic groups are concentrated in the lowest paid and most dangerous jobs (McBarnette, 1996). It is suggested that the increased risk of unemployment faced by minorities acts as a disincentive to complaining about work hazards (Davis *et al.*, 1995). Such problems compound existing health inequalities, with these groups suffering from increased mortality from leading causes as well as higher morbidity than white Americans (Fowler and Risner, 1994).

Research in the UK has also explored the links between ethnicity, occupational settings and health risks. For example, a study of home-working by Phizacklea and Wolkowitz (1995) has shown that gender, class and racial discrimination in the labour market are all important factors leading to the concentration of Asian women in the sectors of this marginal workforce with the lowest pay and the poorest conditions. While there has been little research which directly explores occupational health issues for minority ethnic groups, it is noted that these groups are more likely than their white counterparts to be in low paid occupations, to suffer poor working conditions and to be unemployed, all of which are generally associated with ill health (Douglas, 1996).

Science, knowledge and the control of risk within the work environment

Some of the conceptual challenges to conventional notions of work and risk reflect wider debates about the nature of knowledge and the role of science in society. Until relatively recently, scientific knowledge has been held in high esteem with popular faith resting on the belief that science is based on a secure foundation of objective observation and experiment (Chalmers, 1994). The dominant model of scientific knowledge – laboratory based, concerned with identifying cause and effect relationships, guided by experts and value free – has been transposed onto the study of public health. Thus, current models of risk assessment construct risks as purely technical problems to be resolved by the acquisition of scientific information and the application of rational decision-making processes (Gabe, 1995).

The conventional model of science provides the foundation for the discourse of western scientific medicine that has dominated health care for much of the twentieth century. Smith (1981) has demonstrated the ways in which occupational health provision came to be influenced by this discourse which prioritises 'germ theory' with every disease seen to be caused by a specific bacterium or agent (see also Canaan, this volume). For example, the search by doctors for a single clinical 'condition' similar to tuberculosis hampered attempts to diagnose diffuse respiratory conditions labelled 'black lung' among North American miners during the early twentieth century. This monocausal construction of occupational disease came to replace the broader perspective that had characterised medical accounts prior to the establishment of biomedical hegemony.

In the contemporary setting, disciplines such as occupational hygiene, which is concerned with identifying pathogens in the environment, continue to be constructed in relation to these dominant models of science and medicine. Bailey (1995) cites the Institute of Occupational Hygiene which defines the discipline as concerned with:

> The application of technological and managerial principles for the protection of health by the prevention or reduction of risks to health from chemical, biological or physical agents whether the risks are to people at the workplace or outside it. (IOH, 1993, cited in Bailey, 1995, p. 167).

The limitations of this model are acknowledged even by those working within it. Thus Bailey himself goes on to suggest that the use of these principles to set occupational exposure limits often leads to a false sense of security. This is partly because epidemiological calculations of risk cannot be simply transposed onto individuals (Graham, 1996). In the case of occupational asthma for instance, sensitised individuals can suffer attacks triggered by minute amounts of material well below the occupational exposure limit (Bailey, 1995).

This suggests that decisions about such issues as occupational exposure levels and threshold limit values reflect value judgements about acceptable levels of risk and not just the rational application of scientific information. Questions of values and bias feature strongly in critical accounts of policies and provision for health at work. During the 1970s and early 1980s these accounts often focused on the bias of occupational medicine towards dominant economic and class interests in society. For example, Navarro (1981) argues that scientific claims to neutrality obscure the real causes of occupational disease. These are seen to lie in the processes and relations of production. Work hazards are therefore social, collective phenomena reduced by bourgeois scientists to 'natural', individual problems.

Research suggests that occupational health research and practice have indeed frequently served the interests of employers at the expense of workers: by minimising the scale of work-related illness; limiting compensation costs; prioritising the maintenance of production over the protection of health; ignoring and devaluing workers' experience of occupational ill health and focusing on individual behaviour in explaining work-related illness (Weindling, 1985). More recently, official bodies have been accused of promulgating exposure limits, for example in relation to asbestos, known for many years to be inadequate (Egilman and Reinert, 1995). The scientific establishment has also been accused of ignoring evidence about the occupational and environmental causes of diseases such as breast cancer, focusing exclusively on individual factors such as family history, hormonal factors and dietary fat (Epstein, 1994).

The scientific discourse is seen in some accounts as limiting rather than enhancing knowledge about the work environment (Sass, 1995). Further:

> The scientific approach has not acted as a neutral arbiter of concerns identified by workers, and has permitted employers to turn to varied and diverse professionals for settling work environment disputes. (Sass, 1996, p. 356)

However, as Harrison (1995) suggests, occupational health politics cannot be interpreted simply as a struggle between capital and labour. This perspective does not adequately examine the role of the state and fails to consider the extent to which gender as well as class relations have influenced knowledge about the effects of work on health. In her research on women's work and health in late nineteenth- and early twentieth-century Britain, Harrison reveals a number of paradoxes that have hindered attempts to understand occupational illness and address unhealthy working conditions. During this period notions of danger and female susceptibility were used to exclude women from certain sectors of the workforce. However, factory reformers were more concerned with the threat posed by women's employment to their reproductive and domestic roles, and therefore to the perceived health of the nation, than to the health of women themselves:

> The identification of specific 'dangers' to women who worked would then become a powerful reinforcement of the idea that women should not be working at all. (Harrison, 1996, p. 55)

Harrison suggests that this focus on the special susceptibility of women involved in the 'dangerous trades' caused the dangers to men in these trades to be overlooked and more general occupational health problems in women's employment to be ignored.

Contemporary debates about the production of occupational health knowledge continue to highlight issues of bias. For example, it has been demonstrated that occupational health research is still not gender neutral (OECD, 1993) with differences between men and women often ignored (Lagerlof, 1997). Indeed, women are often excluded from occupational health research altogether because it is assumed that their work is not dangerous, while measures of risk reflect male working patterns and conditions (Messing et al., 1993 a and b; see also Messing, this volume). This problem is often reflected in policy where the male is taken to be the ergonomic norm influencing the design of tools and protective equipment (Quinn et al., 1995).

Epidemiological bias also affects other groups of workers. Davis et al. (1995) highlight the ways in which contemporary research practices result in a lack of data concerning the occupational health status of minority ethnic groups. For example, researchers often choose to focus on whites in the interests of securing more even national comparisons, and when ethnicity is included as a variable in project design it is often ignored in the analysis of study results.

These perspectives call into question the ability of expert-driven scientific and technical strategies to measure and control occupational risks. According to Beck (1992) science is itself part of the problem, with scientific and technological developments generating incalculable unforeseen hazards in what is termed 'risk society'. The traditional assumptions of regulatory politics are inadequate for addressing these risks which span dimensions of time and geographical space. Instead, Beck calls for a reflexive critique of science along the lines of that described by Lash and Wynne (1992) as already operative within the Green movement and among the lay public.

The differences between scientific and lay assessment of risk are explored by Grinyer (1995) in a UK study of health workers' responses to work related risk of HIV infection. She suggests that lay perspectives come closer than scientific discourse to reflecting the complex nature of risk in the work environment. For example, lay perspectives take into account the social dimensions of risk, as is demonstrated in the following quote from a midwife in the study:

> We know that the fact that our patients are on the maternity ward means that they are sexually active, and we know that some of them might be HIV positive, but we'd rather put the patient before the risk. So we don't want to wear goggles and masks while attending women in labour. (cited in Grinyer, 1995, p. 44)

This multidimensional assessment of risk is judged against the comparatively naive insistence of managers, claiming the authority of scientific opinion, that workers need simple information and advice about risk reduction.

These accounts all point towards a call for greater humility in scientific research as well as the need to integrate scientific and lay perspectives on risk. While they recognise that knowledge about risk is shaped by social and cultural processes as well as economic interests, they share a belief that science can be reformed and its methods improved in order to achieve a closer understanding of the work environment.

More radically, some scholars (Armstrong, 1983; Fox, 1993 and also this volume) reject the possibility of achieving unmediated knowledge of the world. This perspective builds on the claim by phenomenologists that human culture is constructed and knowable only through language. However, since language represents the world imperfectly it is argued that it is never possible to reach a perfect understanding of the true essence of things. This perspective points towards the power of discourse to shape perceptions of the world together with the possibilities for action. Hence, it demands that those involved in producing occupational health research be reflexive, recognising the possible impact of their definitions and silences (Fox, 1995; see also Wilton, this volume).

This perspective emphasises the contingent nature of knowledge whether derived from conventional or critical sources and for some leads inevitably to relativism. If one truth is as good as any other how are we to judge competing information and research about the work environment? Others would argue that it highlights the need to make values, goals and assumptions more explicit in the production of knowledge about the relationship between work, risk and health.

The politics of occupational health

The conceptual problems which limit the scope of knowledge about work and risk also impact upon policies and provision for addressing unhealthy working conditions. The control of occupational risk is further complicated by the fact that such risks are increasingly global in origin. There is an increasing need for international perspectives and strategies in this field. While some are pessimistic about the prospect of global regulation, others have argued for increased cooperation between countries in the development of knowledge and the application of controls (Johanning *et al.*, 1994); and for stronger international links between workers and activists (see Pickvance, this volume).

While the ultimate causes of many work-related health problems are global, local differences in regulatory policies can make a significant impact on the health of workers. During the 1980s, for example, the UK government adopted a particularly hostile stance toward occupational health issues: reducing the resources available to regulatory agencies; promoting a philosophy of deregulation; and resisting EU directives (Watterson, 1994 and this volume; see also Pickvance, this volume). It has been argued that these policies contributed directly to the UK's relatively poor record on manufacturing accidents, with significant growth in these documented among some sectors of the workforce such as the self-employed (Tombs, 1996; see also Nichols, this volume).

International strategies for addressing unhealthy working conditions need to recognise conflicting as well as common interests of workers in different countries. For example, workers in industrial societies may benefit from the transfer of risks to poorer countries resulting from increased international economic activity. However, such gains may be short term, offset by the increasing concentration of economic power within multinational companies at the cost of local industries, and the consequent weakening of local labour movements (Greenlund and Elling, 1995). In the long term increasing workplace democracy and workers' power in both industrial and underdeveloped countries are likely to bring more significant improvements to working conditions and health.

Yet the fragmentation of local labour markets and the breakdown of traditional forms of labour organisation, evidenced by declining trade union membership and a shift away from corporatist strategies of economic management, represent increasing problems for workers seeking to improve the working environment and influence occupational health and safety provision. In some instances, the reduced capacity of workers to influence policies through traditional means has led to new forms of activism. For example, outreach work and community campaigns have led to increased organisation around issues of pay and conditions among homeworkers in several countries including Italy, Australia and India. Similarly, in North America, innovative campaigns to build alliances with consumers by developing a union label for use in the fashion industry have been documented (National Group on Homeworking, 1996).

While there are powerful trends towards disempowerment of workers at local level, trends towards greater participation and demands for the democratisation of work have been documented in many parts of the world (see Loewenson *et al.*, this volume). These have led to the growth of participatory research which is seen as part of a process through which new forms of knowledge and change can be achieved. Participatory research builds on the values and insights of popular epidemiology which has grown as a result of increasing public distrust of conventional science and technology (Brown, 1995). In contrast with traditional epidemiology, popular epidemiology is not presented as a value-free enterprise. For example, in the establishment of standards of proof needed for the identification of hazards and the setting of exposure limits, errors on the side of caution in protecting health are preferred to those that protect production or conserve resources. Popular epidemiology examines a wide range of connections between disease and exposure rather than confining investigation to single-exposure disease pairs.

Finally, popular epidemiology draws on people's personal illness narratives rather than dismissing these as misguided and erroneous. Similarly, participatory research in occupational health shifts control of the research process away from professionals to those who actually experience work-related health problems.

The growth of new employment forms means that traditional assumptions about health and safety regulation and management may no longer hold. Many of these approaches have been developed in the context of large companies with paternalistic traditions of occupational welfare, and are unlikely to extend to the growing numbers of self-employed and those working in small businesses. Research has shown that attitudes to health and safety in small firms are different to those in large companies with established safety records and practices. For example, in a Canadian study, Eakin (1992) found that most small business owners accepted the work environment as given and did not see health and safety issues as significant. Employers did not see themselves as having legitimate authority to intervene in matters of health which were seen only to reflect employees' personal behaviour.

Changing patterns of health and risk have led some commentators to question the types of occupational health provision currently available. These take different forms but they are often dominated by employers and are therefore limited in what they are likely to achieve for workers (Pickvance, 1996). While employers might be motivated to comply with health and safety regulations in order to avoid litigation, they are more likely to support health activities which strengthen management and control functions than those aimed at preventing, recognising and providing rehabilitation for work-related ill health (Daykin, 1998). Alternative models have been put forward including forms of group and community provision that currently exist in some European states (Hughes and Rautenberg, 1995; Pickvance, 1996 and this volume). Supporters of these new approaches have stressed the importance of multidisciplinary services in response to changing patterns of work-related ill health.

In some countries, particularly the USA, there is a range of fairly well established employee assistance and wellness programmes. Interest in workplace health promotion as a strategy for improving workers' health and wellbeing is also growing in other industrial countries (Wynne, 1992; Sanders, 1993). Workplace health promotion initiatives do not necessarily focus upon occupational hazards and risks. Instead, they may concentrate on employees' lifestyles and behaviour, offering services such as smoking cessation and counselling as well as exercise and fitness programmes. Yet lifestyles and behaviour may themselves be work related, as work can affect health in both direct and indirect ways (Harvey, 1988). For example, occupational stress and boredom are known to contribute to increased alcohol consumption and liver cirrhosis in a range of manual jobs (Leigh and Jiang, 1993). Behavioural factors may also interact with occupational risks, compounding ill health. For example, research in Norway found that active and passive smoking exerted a combined influence, increasing the risk of lung cancer among waitresses (Kjaerheim and Andersen, 1994).

Hence, workplace health promotion may offer a means of addressing broad problems of work-related illness. However, in drawing attention to workers' habits and lifestyles there is a danger that hazards within the work environment may be ignored and the victims of work-related ill health blamed for their conditions (Watterson, 1986; Daykin, 1990, 1998). Further, the expansion of workplace health promotion raises ethical problems. Conrad and Walsh (1992) have suggested that such programmes are linked to emerging forms of social control, extending employer jurisdiction into the lifestyle of the worker and heralding new forms of employment discrimination.

Drawing on the work of Foucault (1973, 1979), commentators have highlighted the regulatory impact of some health promotion strategies which are seen as belonging to a growing number of technologies of medical surveillance (Armstrong, 1995; Lupton, 1995). This perspective leads to a critical view of many forms of health care as underlining the power and authority of experts and professionals at the expense of recipients. It need not lead to impotence and inaction, however. Fox (1995 and this volume) suggests that practices of control which establish the authority of the knower by disciplining the subjectivies of the cared for can be resisted. They can also be opposed by alternative approaches that celebrate difference and choice.

These insights lead inevitably to scepticism about calls for the straightforward expansion of occupational health provision and regulation. The complex and profoundly political nature of the debate about work and health is further revealed in a number of paradoxes. For example, in the UK, interest in workplace health promotion has increased at the same time as traditional forms of occupational health provision and regulation have declined (see Pickvance this volume). The growth of workplace health promotion does not therefore reflect a broader interest in the health-damaging effects of work but is in fact part of a more general trend away from curative, hospital-based medicine. It is in response to this latter trend that critics have drawn attention to the regulatory impact of all health services. Yet threats to working conditions and health have taken the form of deregulation and not overregulation of health and safety (see Nichols; Watterson and Pickvance, this volume). These policies have been implemented even as some types of health surveillance activity within the workplace have increased. Hence, theories are needed which build upon general critiques of health care but at the same time recognise the specific problems of the relationships between work, risk and health.

These trends and themes are discussed in the contributions that follow. The first four chapters address the implications of changing conditions and definitions of work for the study of occupational health. Lesley Doyal begins by exploring the impact of domestic labour, arguing that although household work takes up a major part of many women's lives, little is known about its effects on health. This is because its low status and invisibility have distracted attention away from possible hazards. She suggests that research in this area is needed to inform the development of gender-sensitive health promotion policies. Such research needs to take account of both similarities and differences in women's experience of household labour and to focus on the links between different dimensions of domestic life.

This is followed by Sarah Payne's chapter which argues that current understanding of mental health in employment is limited by a failure adequately to conceptualise the links between paid and unpaid work. Issues such as control and autonomy, as well as security and insecurity, are generally recognised as significant for the mental health of the employed as well as the unemployed. She argues that a new model is needed which incorporates these factors into an account of the totality of people's lives, including their experience of informal and invisible work. The links between paid and unpaid work are also discussed by Liz Lloyd in her chapter on the occupational hazards facing carers in both paid and unpaid settings. While the hazards may be the same in each of these, the problems of invisibility and lack of regulation of unpaid caring are made clear.

In the next chapter, Graham Scambler and Annette Scambler take up the issue of health and work in the sex industry, arguing that conventional understandings of this area are flawed. They challenge the assumption that women sex workers are passive victims of circumstances and purveyors of disease. The health risks faced by female sex workers, including HIV and sexually transmitted infections, drug use, injury and abuse are examined and a range of health promotion strategies explored.

The next chapter, by Theo Nichols, focuses on recent changes within more traditional forms of paid employment in the formal sector. Conventional explanations of industrial injury are criticised in this chapter which develops a sociological explanation of injury causation, mainly with respect to manufacturing. A discussion of investment-based productivity serves to remind us that technology can make for improvements in safety, a point reinforced by a comparison of coal mining in the UK and in a less developed country, Turkey.

The remaining chapters all explore in various ways the production and reproduction of concepts and knowledge about health and work. First, Andrew Watterson explores some of the reasons why current knowledge about work-related ill health is inadequate. Occupational disease recognition is influenced by underlying economic conditions, with workers facing disincentives to report ill health during times of insecure employment. Social relations are also a powerful influence with little action taken to address occupational diseases perceived to affect only those in lower socioeconomic groups. Watterson proposes a socioparticipative model of occupational health policy as an alternative to current science and expert-led initiatives.

Karen Messing then examines gender bias in occupational health research. She argues that current measures of risk overlook many dimensions of women's work, introducing some of the alternative indicators developed in Quebec that do take these dimensions into account. Her overall criticism is that mainstream science and policy are still a long way from addressing enduring patterns of gender inequality.

The next chapter by Joyce Canaan also explores the limitations of current scientific discourse, in relation to the growing incidence of repetitive strain injury (RSI). The crude separation of physical and psychological causes, and the biological reductionism which has dominated this debate are seen as unhelpful. Not only do these factors act as a barrier to an integrated understanding of this problem, but they also serve to undermine the accounts of victims, discrediting their quests for recognition, treatment and/or compensation.

This is followed by Ruth Pinder's contribution which draws on an ethnographic study of disabled people's experience in the workplace to show that the boundaries between wellness, illness and disablement are not as clear as they might first appear. She questions the belief that discrimination at work can be prevented simply by the imposition of external rules and structures. While these are clearly important, attention also needs to be paid to the ways in which individuals have continually to negotiate complex and shifting boundaries, identities and moral evaluations.

The social construction of occupational hazards is also discussed by Tamsin Wilton in her chapter on risk discourses and their construction of HIV and AIDS. She suggests that conventional notions of risk and what constitutes an occupation are inadequate for dealing with the complexities of HIV risk. At the same time she warns against the straightforward extension of professional activity in this area, pointing towards the likely impact of such expansion for regulation and control. Instead, she recommends that those involved recognise and take responsibility for the constitutive power of discourses of occupational health and illness.

The discussion of risk discourses continues in the chapter by Nick Fox. This offers a postmodern perspective in which both risks and hazards are seen as social fabrications, grounded in various claims to knowledge and authority. Fox examines the effects of this process of social construction, in which 'riskiness' and therefore moral responsibility are attributed to human behaviour, on individual subjectivities. He also argues that it is possible to resist this process, and he asserts the positive potential of choices and risks in the right circumstances.

The final two chapters explore policies and strategies for addressing occupational risks and improving occupational health services. In his chapter, Simon Pickvance discusses five areas of policy and practice: prevention; regulation and enforcement; rehabilitation; compensation; and research. Drawing on his experience with a community-based occupational health service in the UK, he highlights the importance of local policy and action in the context of increased globalisation of occupational risk.

The last chapter, by Rene Loewenson, Asa Laurell and Christer Hogstedt, explores the contribution that participatory research can make to the understanding of occupational risk. Drawing on examples from Sweden, Zimbabwe, Italy and Latin America, they argue that participatory research not only generates new forms of knowledge, but also serves as a force for change in the field of occupational health and in the broader process of democratisation of the work environment.

Acknowledgements

I am grateful to Lesley Doyal for her incisive comments in discussion of the issues raised in this chapter as well as her rigorous reading of an earlier draft. Thanks are also due to Joyce Canaan, Theo Nichols, Ruth Pinder and Tamsin Wilton for their helpful suggestions and to Jenny Dafforn for her help in preparing the manuscript.

References

Armstrong, D. (1983) *Political Anatomy of the Body: Medical Knowledge in Britain in the Twentieth Century.* Cambridge: Cambridge University Press.
Armstrong, D. (1995) 'The rise of surveillance medicine', *Sociology of Health and Illness*, **17**(3): 393–404.
Artus, K. (1995) 'Diseases of occupations' in S. Pantry (ed.), *Occupational Health.* London: Chapman & Hall.
Bailey, S. (1995) 'Occupational hygiene' in S. Pantry (ed.), *Occupational Health.* London: Chapman & Hall.

Bartley, M. and Owen, C. (1996) 'Relation between socioeconomic status, employment and health during economic change, 1973–93', *BMJ*, **313** (24 August): 445–9.

Beck, U. (1992) *Risk Society: Towards a New Modernity*. London: Sage.

Berger, P.L. and Luckman, T. (1967) *The Social Construction of Reality*. London: Allen Lane, Penguin.

Brewster, C., Mayne, L. and Tregaskis, O. (1997) 'Flexible working in Europe: a review of the evidence', *Management International Review*, Special Issue, (1): 85–103.

Brown, P. (1995) 'Popular epidemiology, toxic waste and social movements' in J. Gabe (ed.), *Medicine, Health and Risk. Sociological Approaches*. Oxford: Blackwell.

Cameron, A. (1995) 'Work and change in industrial society: a sociological perspective' in M. Bamford (ed.), *Work and Health: An Introduction to Occupational Health Care*. London: Chapman & Hall.

Chalmers, A.F. (1994) *What Is This Thing Called Science?* Buckingham: Open University Press.

Conrad, P. and Walsh, D.C. (1992) 'The new corporate health ethic: lifestyle and the social control of work', *International Journal of Health Services*, **22**(1): 89–111.

Davis, M.E., Rowland, A.S., Walker, B. Jr. and Kidd Taylor, A. (1995) 'Minority workers' in B.S. Levy and D.H. Wegman (eds), *Occupational Health: Recognising and Preventing Work-Related Disease*. London: Little, Brown.

Daykin, N. (1990) 'Health and work in the 1990s: towards a new perspective' in P. Abbott and G. Payne (eds), *New Directions in the Sociology of Health*. London: Falmer.

Daykin, N. (1998) 'Workplace health promotion: benefit or burden to low paid workers', *Critical Public Health*, **8**(2): 153–66.

Dodier, N. (1985) 'Social uses of illness at the workplace: sick leave and moral evaluation', *Social Science and Medicine*, **20**(2): 123–8.

Douglas, J. (1996) 'Developing with Black and minority ethnic communities, health promotion strategies which address social inequalities' in P. Bywaters and E. McLeod (eds), *Working for Equality in Health*. London: Routledge.

Doyal, L. (1995) *What Makes Women Sick? Gender and the Political Economy of Health*. London: Macmillan.

Eakin, J.M. (1992) 'Leaving it up to the workers: sociological perspective on the management of health and safety in small workplaces', *International Journal of Health Services*, **22**(4): 689–704.

Egilman, D.S. and Reinert, A.A. (1995) 'The origin and development of the asbestos threshold limit value: scientific indifference and corporate influence', *International Journal of Health Services*, **25**(4): 667–96.

Elling, R.H. (1981) 'Industrialisation and Occupational Health in Underdeveloped countries' in V. Navarro and D.M. Berman (eds), *Health and Work under Capitalism: An International Perspective*. New York: Baywood.

Epstein, S.S. (1994) 'Environmental and occupational pollutants are avoidable causes of breast cancer', *International Journal of Health Services*, **24**(1): 145–50.

Fatusi, A. and Erhabor, G. (1996) 'Occupational health status of sawmill workers in Nigeria', *Journal of the Royal Society of Health*, **116**(4): 232–6.

Floyd, M., Povall, M. and Watson, G. (1994) (eds) *Mental Health at Work*. London: Jessica Kingsley.

Foucault, M. (1973) *The Birth of the Clinic: An Archaeology of Medical Perception*. New York: Vintage Books.

Foucault, M. (1979) *Discipline and Punish. The Birth of the Prison*. London: Penguin.

Fowler, B.A. and Risner, P.B. (1994) 'A health promotion program evaluation in a minority industry', *ABNF Journal*, May–June, **5**(3): 72–6.

Fox, N. (1993) *Postmodernism: Sociology and Health*. Buckingham: Open University.

Fox, N. (1995) 'Postmodern perspectives on care: the vigil and the gift', *Critical Social Policy*, **44/45** (Autumn): 107–25.

Gabe, J. (1995) 'Health, medicine and risk: the need for a sociological approach' in J. Gabe (ed.), *Medicine, Health and Risk: Sociological Approaches*. Oxford: Blackwell.

Graham, H. (1996) 'Research on women and poverty: trends and future directions' in N. Daykin and L. Lloyd (eds), *Researching Women, Gender and Health*. Report of a conference, UWE, 17 June 1995. Bristol: Bristol Women and Health Research Group/UWE, Faculty of Health and Social Care, Glenside Campus, B516 1DD.

Green, J. (1992) 'The medico–legal production of fatal accidents', *Sociology of Health and Illness*, **14**(3): 373–89.

Greenlund, K.J. and Elling, R.H. (1995) 'Capital sectors and worker's health and safety in the United States', *International Journal of Health Services*, **25**(1): 101–16.

Grinyer, A. (1995) 'Risk, the real world and naive sociology: perceptions of risk from occupational injury in the health service' in J. Gabe (ed.), *Medicine, Health and Risk: Sociological Approaches*. Oxford: Blackwell.

Harrison, B. (1995) 'The politics of occupational ill-health in late nineteenth century Britain: the case of the match making industry', *Sociology of Health and Illness*, **17**(1): 20–41.

Harrison, B. (1996) *Not Only the 'Dangerous Trades' Women's Work and Health in Britain 1880–1914*. London: Taylor & Francis.

Harvey, S. (1988) *Just an Occupational Hazard? Policies for Health at Work*. London: King's Fund Institute.

Heaney, C.A., Israel, B.A. and House, J.S. (1994) 'Chronic job insecurity among automobile workers: effects on job satisfaction and health', *Social Science and Medicine*, **38**(10): 1431–7.

Hughes, M. and Rautenberg, S. (1995) *Occupational Health Services in Denmark: A Model for the UK?*. Discussion Paper (unpublished) Leeds Occupational Health Project, March.

Johanning, E., Goldberg, M. and Kim, R. (1994) 'Asbestos hazard evaluation in South Korean Textile Production', *International Journal of Health Services*, **24**(1): 131–44.

Karasek, R. and Theorell, T. (1990) *Healthy Work: Stress, Productivity and the Reconstruction of Working Life*. Basic Books: New York.

Kjaerheim, K. and Andersen, A. (1994) 'Cancer incidence among waitresses in Norway', *Cancer Causes and Control*, **5**: 31–6.

Lagerlof, E. (1997) 'European women – their health, safety and working conditions'. Unpublished Conference Paper, First international course on

Gender, Work and Psychosocial Health, Hotel Eckero, Aland, Finland, 9–13 June.

Lash, S. and Wynne, B. (1992) 'Introduction' in U. Beck, *Risk Society: Towards a New Modernity*. London: Sage.

Leigh, J.P. and Jiang, W.Y. (1993) 'Liver cirrhosis deaths within occupations and industries in the California Mortality Study', *Addiction*, **88**: 767–79.

Levenstein, C., Wooding, J. and Rosenberg, B. (1995) The social context of occupational health' in B.S. Levy and D.H. Wegman (eds), *Occupational Health: Recognising and Preventing Work-Related Disease*. Boston/New York/Toronto/London: Little, Brown.

Levy, B.S. and Wegman, D.H. (1995) 'Occupational health in the global context: an American perspective' in B.S.Levy and D.H. Wegman (eds), *Occupational Health: Recognising and Preventing Work-Related Disease*. Boston/New York/Toronto/London: Little, Brown.

Lupton, D. (1995) *The Imperative of Health: Public Health and the Regulated Body*. London: Sage.

McBarnette, L.S. (1996) 'African American women' in M. Bayne-Smith (ed.), *Race, Gender, and Health*. London: Sage.

Messing, K., Doniol-Shaw, G. and Haentjens, C. (1993a) 'Sugar and spice and everything nice: health effects of the sexual division of labour among train cleaners', *International Journal of Health Services*, **23**(1): 133–46.

Messing, K., Dumais, L. and Romito, P. (1993b) 'Prostitutes and chimney sweeps both have problems: towards full integration of both sexes in the study of occupational health', *Social Science and Medicine*, **36**(1): 47–55.

National Group on Homeworking (1996) Briefing Paper No 1.

Navarro, V. (1981) 'Work, ideology and science: the case of medicine' in V. Navarro and D.M. Berman (eds), *Health and Work under Capitalism: An International Perspective*. New York: Baywood.

Nettleton, S. (1995) *The Sociology of Health and Illness*. Cambridge: Polity.

Nichols, T. (1997) *The Sociology of Industrial Injury*. London: Mansell.

Nichols, T. (1998) 'Review article: health and safety at work' in *Work, Employment and Society*, **12**(2): 367–74.

OECD (1993) 'Women, work and health. Synthesis report of a panel of experts', OCDEIGD (93) 182 Paris.

Packard, R. (1989) 'Industrial production, health and disease in Sub-Saharan Africa', *Social Science and Medicine*, **28**(5): 475–96.

Phizacklea, A. and Wolkowitz, C. (1995) *Homeworking Women: Gender, Racism and Class at Work*. London: Sage.

Pickvance, S. (1996) 'Towards multidisciplinary prevention services', *Occupational Health Review*, (Sept/Oct): 27–32.

Pinder, R. (1995) 'Bringing back the body without the blame?: the experience of ill and disabled people at work', *Sociology of Health and Illness*, **17**(5): 605–31.

Quinn, M.M., Woskie, S.R. and Rosenberg, B.J. (1995) 'Women and work' in B. Levy and D.H. Wegman (eds), *Occupational Health: Recognising and Preventing Work-Related Disease*. Boston/New York/Toronto/London: Little, Brown.

Sanders, D. (1993) *Workplace Health Promotion: A Review of the Literature*. Oxford: Oxford Regional Health Authority.

Sass, R. (1995) 'A conversation about the work environment', *International Journal of Health Services*, **25**(1): 117–28.

Sass, R. (1996) 'A strategic response to the occupational health establishment', *International Journal of Health Services*, **26**(2): 355–70.

Smith, B.E. (1981) 'Black lung: the social production of disease' in V. Navarro and D.N. Berman (eds), *Health and Work under Capitalism: An International Perspective*. New York: Baywood.

Takala, J. (1995) 'Worldwide view of occupational health and safety' in S. Pantry (ed.), *Occupational Health*. London: Chapman & Hall.

Tancred, P. (1995) 'Women's work: a challenge to the sociology of work', *Gender, Work and Organisation*, **2**(1): 11–20.

Tombs, S. (1996) 'Injury, death and the deregulation fetish: the politics of occupational safety regulation in UK manufacturing industries', *International Journal of Health Services*, **26**(2): 309–29.

Virtanen, P. (1994) '"An epidemic of good health" at the workplace', *Sociology of Health and Illness*, **16**(3): 394–401.

Watterson, A. (1986) 'Occupational health and illness: the politics of hazard education' in S. Rodmell and A. Watt (eds), *The Politics of Health Education*. London: Routledge & Kegan Paul.

Watterson, A. (1994) 'Threats to health and safety in the workplace in Britain', *BMJ*, **308** (30 April): 1115–16.

Weindling, P. (ed.) (1985) *The Social History of Occupational Health*. London: Croom Helm.

Whittaker, D. and Hart, D.G. (1996) 'Research note: managing risks: the social organisation of indoor sex work', *Sociology of Health and Illness*, **18**(3): 399–414.

Wilkinson, R.G. (1996) *Unhealthy Societies: The Afflictions of Inequality*. London: Routledge.

Williams, J. (1996) 'Stress: a guide for organisations', *Occupational Health*, (July): 240–2.

Williams, N. (1995) 'The occupational health aspects of working from home', *Occupational Health*, (March): 95–6.

Wynne, R. (1992) *Innovative Workplace Actions for Health: An Overview of the Situation in Seven EC Countries*. Dublin: European Foundation for the Improvement of Living and Working Conditions.

1 WOMEN AND DOMESTIC LABOUR: SETTING A RESEARCH AGENDA

Lesley Doyal

A key theme of this volume concerns the problems of conventional definitions of work that limit the parameters of occupational health research and practice. This theme is addressed in the following chapter that focuses on the labour carried out within households. This is rarely seen as 'real' work and has received very little attention from those concerned with occupational health and safety. It is also the most 'gendered' form of labour, since domestic tasks are identified as 'female' across the vast majority of societies. The nature of this work has certain similarities wherever it is being performed but it is also shaped in profound ways by cultural, economic and social circumstances. This chapter offers a research agenda for enhancing our understanding of the impact of domestic work in a range of social settings on those (predominantly) women who carry it out. It also provides some preliminary thoughts on the implications of research findings for broadening the scope of occupational health and safety policy.

Introduction

For many women domestic labour takes up a major part of their lives but we know relatively little about how this affects their health. There are two major reasons for this ignorance. The first is the social and physical invisibility of household work. Its location behind closed doors and its low status have distracted attention from possible hazards in the work itself. If domestic labour is 'natural ' for women then surely it is 'good' for them is the implicit assumption. In recent years this pattern has begun to change as many women have 'come out' and are talking in public about aspects of their lives that had previously remained private. But despite these revelations our knowledge remains very partial, reflecting the multidimensional and fragmented nature of the work itself.

'Work' is a complex activity which is difficult to analyse even when it is formally defined and contained within a place of paid employment, such as a shop or a factory. Tasks carried out in the domestic arena can be even more varied, making it difficult to estimate their impact on wellbeing. Around the world, household labour has certain similarities. It is usually unpaid, low in status, has no time limits and offers relatively few opportunities for self-development. Yet there are also major differences in both the work and the working conditions of different groups of women around the world and studies need to reflect this diversity. Research into the health implications of women's domestic labour is rarely funded and can be challenging to carry out but it must be undertaken if we are to have an accurate knowledge base for the development of gender-sensitive health promotion policies.

In all countries, women have the primary responsibility for household labour – both for 'caring for' others and also 'caring about ' them. However, the content of this work will vary in different historical periods and social settings. Today the most obvious divisions in domestic work can be found between those women in rich countries who are relatively affluent and the millions who try to survive in either rural or urban poverty in other parts of the world. In the developed countries, women's responsibilities as 'housewives' and carers means ensuring their own and their family's physical and psychological wellbeing through the translation of money and other resources into items for daily consumption. Cooking, cleaning, washing and the provision of emotional support all come into this category of activity which for many will be combined with paid work.

Most women in poor countries have to carry out the same duties but often under much more onerous conditions. In addition, many have to do heavy labour, working directly on their immediate material environment to ensure that adequate resources are available to meet their family's most basic needs. They may have to grow and process food, for instance, as well as collecting fuel and water. In this setting it is often very difficult to separate household labour, subsistence agriculture and

income-generating work in the informal sector. For the women themselves both the physical and the psychological burdens are often
extremely heavy, yet the health effects of their work go unremarked.

This chapter sets out a framework for exploring these effects across a
variety of social settings. It will give a brief account of what is known
and not known about the impact of women's domestic work on their
health and suggest some of the methods that need to be used if we are
to find out more. It will demonstrate the need for a broad range of disciplinary perspectives as well as a variety of data-collection techniques if
a coherent account of the relationship between women's domestic
work and their wellbeing is to be achieved. Five major issues will be
identified as central to this research agenda:

- Our first concern must be to understand the structural patterns of
  women's domestic lives. Just as traditional occupational health
  research might begin by exploring women's position in the labour
  market so there is a need to explore the sizes and types of households
  women live in and the range of tasks they perform in those settings.
- As well as learning more about the nature of household work we
  also need to explore the physical hazards it can pose. The home needs
  to be recognised as a workplace like any other and the material risks
  it presents for those working inside it need to be identified and
  acknowledged.
- At the same time, the concept of risk has to be extended to look at the
  psychological hazards of being a woman worker in the household
  environment. Just as the scope of occupational health research is
  being expanded to include factors such as stress in working life, so we
  have to explore the ways in which unpaid and low status work may
  be damaging to a woman's mental health.
- There is also an urgent need to put violence on the agenda as a
  serious risk faced by millions of women in their own households.
  This is a public health hazard which affects women throughout the
  world and more research is needed to determine the most effective
  strategies for ameliorating its effects on both physical and mental
  health.
- Finally, we need to explore in much greater depth the pattern of
  gender inequalities in the distribution of resources within
  households. We need to have a clearer understanding of how
  women are emotionally and materially rewarded for the work they
  do and whether those rewards are adequate to maintain their
  health.

Measuring and mapping household labour

Information on some of the most basic aspects of women's lives is to be found in official statistics, both those collected in individual countries and also those collated by international organisations such as the United Nations (UN, 1991; UNDP, 1995). However more work is needed to draw out the implications of these data for women's labour and for their wellbeing. The quantification of their workload, for example, can be derived in part from data on family size and structure, including the number of older people and disabled people in a population and the availability of services to care for them. The number of one-parent families is an especially significant indicator since in these settings women are likely to be the only breadwinner and the sole carer.

In the USA, more than a third of households are headed by women, while in Botswana, as in many other parts of Africa, that figure is as high as 45 per cent (UN, 1991). We know that these households are economically disadvantaged and that the women involved often have to take on a punishing burden of work. However, they may avoid other risks such as physical and emotional abuse. More qualitative studies are therefore needed to determine the health-promoting or damaging features of different types of households. Research of this kind poses considerable methodological challenges with a complex set of variables to be investigated, but it is an important area of work as traditional patterns of family life are transformed in so many parts of the world (Bortolaia Silva, 1996).

Demographic statistics can give us some indication of the volume of household work but it will of course be only a partial picture unless we can also look inside the family to determine in more detail both the type of work being done and its allocation between different household members. The nature of the work is especially important when we are making cross-cultural comparisons. As we have seen, in the developed countries 'housework' and caring are relatively limited activities compared with the burden of work in many of the world's poorest countries where women have to grapple directly with the natural world if they are to provide what is necessary for their families (Doyal, 1995). Thus the health impact of household work needs to be much more carefully delineated in different social and economic contexts.

But even when we know the nature of the work, we need to go further, to discover who is actually doing it. There is a general acceptance that women bear the heaviest burdens but this needs to be more carefully documented. More reliable data are needed on variations in the division of domestic labour both in the volume of work done and also in the allocation of different tasks. Accurate information about household functioning can be extremely difficult to obtain especially on topics as potentially sensitive as who does what. However, the development of techniques such as time use analysis is beginning to give new insights on gender and age divisions in the allocation of household work (UN, 1991).

Physical hazards of household labour

Having identified the nature and volume of the domestic work women carry out, we then need to look much more carefully at the physical hazards these labours may pose for them. Many of the more traditional methods of research used by health and safety practitioners can be of value here. However, they have rarely been used in the domestic setting, presumably because of the continuing tendency to assume that what goes on inside it is not real work.

One of the first questions needing careful attention is the definition of the workplace itself. We can start with the 'home' – the physical building in which women do much of their unpaid work. The nature of this structure will obviously have a major impact on both the volume of their labour and the risks they are likely to incur and those with the least resources are likely to be at the greatest risk (McCarthy et al., 1985; Hyndman, 1990). However, for many women their domestic labour spreads well beyond the physical confines of the house.

In a recent article Kettel has emphasised the need to explore both the biophysical and the social environments in which women do their work. She talks about the importance of understanding the 'natural and constructed life spaces within which women carry out their gender-based involvement as domestic workers, producers and income earners' (Kettel, 1996, p. 1369). We can illustrate these points in more detail through looking at two examples of physical hazards: damage caused by the lifting of heavy weights and exposure to toxic substances.

Women's domestic labour can require them to lift weights several times greater than the limits that would be set if they were formally employed. This is especially true in those parts of the world where they are responsible for water and fuel collection, much of which will have to be continued late into pregnancy. There have been few systematic attempts to explore the health consequences of these practices but anecdotal evidence indicates that serious back injuries, uterine prolapses and miscarriage are not uncommon (Chatterjee, 1991; Rodda, 1991; Sims, 1994). We need to know much more about these problems since ergonomic techniques could be of great value if used appropriately.

There is also growing evidence that because of their domestic responsibilities, women are exposed to chemicals from which they might be protected in employment (Dowie *et al.*, 1982; Rosenberg, 1984). To take one recent example, it is now evident that many are exposed to serious pollutants because of the time spent indoors near cooking stoves. This can cause acute bronchitis as well as nasopharyngeal cancer and we need to know more about these extremely damaging effects (Chen *et al.*, 1990; Behera *et al.*, 1991; Norboo *et al.*, 1991; Sims, 1994). The technology exists for the provision of non-polluting stoves and we need to use research findings to try and ensure that those women who need them are able to acquire them.

In many countries both male and female workers have their health protected by regulations limiting the weight they can be expected to lift and the substances they can be exposed to. While these are not always adhered to they do offer some protection, setting out levels of unacceptable risk against which workers can appeal. No such standards exist in the domestic environment and yet, as we have seen, there are similar risks. In the case of both physical hazards and toxic exposure the investigative techniques required to identify them have already been developed. What is needed is a wider acceptance that domestic work can be genuinely hazardous and the devising of regulatory strategies to control this.

In some parts of the world recent research has also identified an entirely new area of risk associated with patterns of domestic labour. This involves the transmission of infectious diseases, especially those related to water and the so-called tropical diseases spread through contact with vectors (Manderson *et al.*, 1993; Rathgeber and Vlassoff, 1993; Vlassoff and Bonilla, 1994). Some aspects of gender socialisation may protect women. In the case of malaria for instance, those women who are required to keep their bodies covered and rarely go out in public appear to have a greater degree of protection from mosquito bites (Reuben, 1993). Other aspects of the gender division of labour have the opposite effect, however.

In most settings, women's responsibilities for household sanitation, clothes washing and some agricultural tasks bring them into contact more often than men with water and with the vectors for some diseases. Diarrhoea, schistosomiasis and malaria all come into this category. In the case of schistosomiasis for example, the numbers of males infected drops after adolescence when they stop playing around water but that of females remains stable as their domestic duties require repeated exposure to the disease-carrying aquatic snails (Michelson, 1993; Sims, 1994).

Psychological risks of domestic work

Any attempt to understand the psychological hazards of work in the home faces complex methodological problems concerning the identification and labelling of mental health and illness. It is well known that national statistics (taken mostly from the developed countries) show an overrepresentation of women in general and 'housewives' in particular in the population defined as 'anxious' and 'depressed' (Dennerstein *et al.*, 1993; Desjarlais *et al.*, 1995). Smaller scale studies are now beginning to show a similar pattern in a wide range of countries (Davis and Guarnaccia, 1989; Chakraborty, 1990; Malik *et al.*, 1992). However, these findings can be difficult to interpret.

What are they really telling us about women's mental wellbeing? Are they simply reflecting women's greater propensity to admit their weakness and possibly to take their emotional problems to a doctor? Are they a result of the tendency of health workers (and others) to assume that women are more likely than men to be psychologically disturbed? Or are they 'real', stemming directly from the particular stresses created in many women's lives by the domestic division of labour? The answer is, probably, all three, but more qualitative research is needed to understand these issues in greater depth. In particular we need a clearer understanding of the different dimensions of household dynamics that are involved in producing these gender differences in mental health.

Issues that need to be disentangled include the relative influences of domestic labour itself – its routine and repetitive character for example – by comparison with its low social status and the failure of many family members to recognise women's contribution to their collective wellbeing. Alongside this we need a better understanding of the impact of 'unequal worth' in family life on women's health. When individuals spend much of their time in a setting where they are seen as less valuable than others, this can affect their wellbeing at a number of different levels.

One aspect of particular concern here is the impact of the sexual division of caring which often gives women responsibility for looking after others but rarely gives them adequate social support in doing so

(Miles, 1988; Belle, 1990). We also need to gain a better understanding of the significance of mothering itself. Although it is clearly the primary emotional experience of many women's lives, recent studies have suggested that it can sometimes be damaging to their health (Romito, 1990).

There are a number of classic studies that have provided an important starting point for this work: Ann Oakley's pioneering studies of British housewives and mothers for example (Oakley, 1974, 1976) and the work done by George Brown and Tyrell Harris on the mental health of working-class women in south London (Brown and Harris, 1978). What these and similar studies have in common is that they are carried out in depth on a relatively small sample. In their different ways they are attempting to look at the many dimensions of women's lives, to explore the meanings they have for the women involved and to assess the implications this may have for their mental health.

Much more research of this kind is needed in very different types of households in different societies if we are to understand the psychological significance of women's domestic work in an appropriately sophisticated way. The work of anthropologists is especially important here, since our current understanding of these issues continues to be based predominantly on the domestic experiences of white women in Britain and the USA. The value of cross-cultural work in this area is evident from a number of recent studies exploring the 'nervous' symptoms commonly reported by 'ordinary' women in so many societies (Davis and Guarnaccia, 1989; Finkler, 1989). These have provided important insights into the relationship between cultural factors and women's material circumstances in the construction of their mental health.

This qualitative approach to the exploration of women's domestic lives has also been valuable in understanding their use and abuse of potentially hazardous substances such as tranquillisers, alcohol and cigarettes (Doyal, 1995). Hilary Graham's work on low income mothers and smoking in the UK is probably one of the best examples because it places what might otherwise be defined as individual moral weakness into a social context where gender divisions are recognised as a significant variable (Graham, 1993). Of course these are not easy research tasks. They require tact, sensitivity and the capacity for flexibility in the development of new methods of investigation. However, it is essential that they are continued if we are to go beyond the superficial in our understanding of the impact of women's domestic work on their choice of unhealthy strategies for coping with the stress in their lives.

Private violence and public health

Moving on to our fourth category of risk, we need to confront a major threat to both the mental and the physical health of millions of women. The fact that violence in included on the research agenda for examining the impact of women's domestic work on their health might at first sight appear paradoxical. The general assumption about families is that they provide a haven from the hazards of the outside world. However, it is becoming increasingly evident that this is often far from the truth. Indeed, women are usually more protected in the public world of work than in the private world of the home. We do not know in precise terms how extensive this problem is and identifying the numbers of women affected is a key part of the research agenda. But we do know that the numbers are large.

In a recent World Development Report, the World Bank estimated that at minimum, rape and domestic violence together are responsible for about 19 per cent of the total disease burden of women aged 15 to 44 in the developed countries and 5 per cent in the developing countries where the burden of other diseases is very much greater (World Bank, 1993). So an important, although difficult, task of researchers in this area is to be more precise about the numbers of women affected and the circumstances under which they are most likely to be threatened. This will necessitate especially sensitive and creative methods, and usually the active involvement of women in the community under review.

We also need to know much more about the effects of violence on women's health. On the face of it these may seem obvious – a battered woman's wounds may be only too visible. However, there is a growing volume of research identifying the longer-term and often more insidious effects violence may have (Heise *et al.*, 1994). Studies have shown for instance, that women who have experienced battering are more likely than others to be depressed and/or to be substance abusers (Andrews and Brown, 1988; Plichta, 1992). They are also at increased risk of committing suicide (Stark and Flitcraft, 1991). The dynamics behind these long-term effects need careful investigation and this will require more collaboration between therapists and those involved in research.

The prevention of domestic violence is an extremely challenging task to which there is no simple answer but researchers have a role here in carrying out rigorous evaluations of the various strategies being adopted around the world. In particular, more work is needed to determine the effectiveness (or otherwise) of counselling designed to reduce the violent behaviour of individual offenders. The findings can then be developed into educational programmes and good practice guidelines to be used by clinicians and others involved in the identification and treatment of the damage wrought by domestic violence.

Who gets what? Gender inequalities in the allocation of household resources

The final item to be placed on this research agenda is the allocation of resources inside families and households. There is an urgent need for more detailed examination of the different types of 'payment' women receive and for an assessment of the degree to which these are appropriate for the maintenance of good health. The rewards paid to workers in employment are very obvious since they come in the form of a wage packet. In the case of domestic labour these links are much less transparent but the effects on health may be even more profound. There is a common sense assumption that households generally try to promote the wellbeing of their members and that resources are distributed equally, or at least according to need. However, recent research has begun to cast doubt on this assumption.

As we have seen, access to the inner workings of households is often very difficult to obtain. Not surprisingly, information about the allocation of resources is especially sensitive but a number of new techniques are beginning to shed light on this important topic (Rogers and Schlossman, 1990; Haddad, 1992). We know that many millions of women around the world continue to be dependent for their survival on what they are given within the household. This includes many of those with large families and many for whom there are major cultural obstacles to work outside the home. Even those in waged work usually receive less than a man in an equivalent position and in some societies they are expected to hand over the money they make to the man of the family. Women's domestic labours are often very demanding especially if they are combined with work outside in either the formal or informal sectors. Yet this is often ignored in determining their access to household resources.

We have seen that non-material rewards such as care and support are often kept from women and that this can have a significant effect on their mental health. The same appears to be true of more visible resources such as money. Although the degree of inequality in income varies markedly between societies, it is evident both in developed societies and in those that are poorer and more intensely patriarchal.

Official statistics give us little help in exploring these issues. This is in part because they give little or no information about the informal sector and also because most data are presented by households, giving almost no idea about the distribution between adults and children and men and women within those households. We therefore have to rely on the new household studies that are being carried out in many parts of the world using a variety of techniques to ensure more accurate recording of income and expenditure and of economic decision making (Haddad *et al.*, 1994). If the links are to be made between relative poverty within the family and overall levels of health, then closer cooperation will be required between epidemiologists and social scientists in the interpretation of complex patterns of social behaviour and their biological outcomes.

Interdisciplinary work of this kind has been developing rapidly in recent years in the area of nutritional anthropology with studies in a number of different countries showing gender bias in the allocation of food and commodities (Messer, 1997). The methodological challenges in this work are significant and the findings are not always consistent. It would be surprising if they were, since both material and cultural differences between societies will affect how resources were allocated. However, a common finding in many parts of the world is that the health of young girls and women is damaged by the fact that they are less adequately nourished and receive less medical care than males in the family.

The most graphic evidence of the effects of this discrimination can be seen in the differential rates of morbidity and mortality found in a number of countries including India, Bangladesh, Nepal, and Peru (Graham, 1997; Miller, 1997). Its overall effects were highlighted by Amartya Sen, the economist, in his discussion of the 'missing millions' of women in parts of Asia (Sen, 1990). These women died prematurely because the social and cultural criteria for the allocation of health promoting resources privileged their fathers, husbands and brothers despite the fact that pregnancy and child bearing often meant that their own need was greater.

Among those women who survive, lack of an adequate diet can cause continuing morbidity and sickness and these gendered inequalities in wellbeing have received increasing attention in recent years. Research is growing especially in the poorest parts of the world where inadequate diets remain common for both sexes but especially for women. The most obvious indicator of this problem is the statistical data published regularly by WHO on the prevalence of anaemia among women of reproductive age.

Recent estimates suggest that 40–50 per cent of women in developing countries and about 10 per cent of those in the industrialised countries are anaemic, with the number rising to more than 50 per cent and 17 per cent respectively among pregnant women (UN, 1991). The prevalence is highest in South Asia (at 80 per cent in some countries) demonstrating the mismatch between women's reproductive health needs and the way resources are often allocated within families. Given their heavy burden of work many are not able to feed themselves sufficiently well to sustain their health, and more detailed analyses are required if the implications of this are to be fully explored.

Here again cooperation is required, this time between nutritionists and social scientists, to try to understand the implications for women's health of gender inequalities in both the division of work and the allocation of household resources. Moreover, such research is not only needed in the world's poorest countries. Even in the UK, with a welfare state that is supposed to provide support from birth to death, research has shown that many women cannot afford a healthy diet during pregnancy (Durward, 1988).

Conclusion

This chapter has offered a framework for carrying out research on the health implications of women's domestic work. This is an important topic, yet it has so far received scant attention. Many feminist researchers have looked at single aspects of women's domestic lives – at housework and depression for example, or gender violence or nutrition. What is needed now is a conceptual framework that brings together our understanding of these very different aspects of women's lives as part of the same reality. This is a challenging task which will necessitate interdisciplinary working and the use of a wide range of methods for data collection and analysis. It will also require an open and participatory approach to those whose private lives will be explored. In undertaking this work we will need to treat the differences between women as seriously as the similarities. In particular, we will need to explore domestic work across the lifecycle so that we can regard the needs of older women as seriously as those of younger women. The aim should be to make both domestic work and waged work healthier for all women and the right kind of research has an important role to play in bringing that about.

Bibliography

Andrews, B. and Brown, G. (1988) 'Violence in the community: a biographical approach', *British Journal of Psychiatry*, **153**: 305–12.

Behera, D., Dash, S. and Yadar, S. (1991) 'Carboxyhaemoglobin in women exposed to different cooking fuels', *Thorax*, **46**: 344–6.

Belle, D. (1990) 'Poverty and women's mental health', *American Psychologist*, **45**: 385–9.

Bortolaia Silva, E. (1996) *Good Enough Mothering? Feminist Perspectives on Late Motherhood*. London: Routledge.

Brown, G. and Harris, T. (1978) *Social Origins of Depression*. London: Tavistock.

Chakraborty, A. (1990) *Social Stress and Mental Health: A Social-psychiatric Field Study of Calcutta*. New Delhi: Sage.

Chatterjee, M. (1991) *Indian Women: Their Health and Productivity*. Washington DC: World Bank.

Chen, B., Hong, C., Pandey, M. and Smith, K. (1990) 'Indoor air pollution in developing countries', *World Health Statistics Quarterly*, **43**: 127–38.

Davis, D. and Guarnaccia, D. (1989) 'Wealth, culture and the nature of nerves: an introduction', *Medical Anthropology*, **11**: 1–13.

Dennerstein, L., Astbury, J. and Morse, C. (1993) *Psychosocial and Mental Health Aspects of Women's Health*. Geneva: WHO.

Desjarlais, R., Eisenberg, L., Good, B. and Kleinman, A. (1995) *World Mental Health: Problems and Priorities in Low-income Countries*. Oxford: Oxford University Press.

Dowie, M., Foster, D., Marshall, C., Weir, D. and King, J. (1982) 'The illusion of safety', *Mother Jones*: 38–48.

Doyal, L. (1995) *What Makes Women Sick: Gender and the Political Economy of Health*. London: Macmillan.

Durward, L. (1988) *Poverty in Pregnancy: The Cost of an Adequate Diet for Pregnant Mothers*. London: Maternity Alliance.

Finkler, K. (1989) 'The universality of nerves', *Health Care for Women International*, **10**(2 and 3): 171–9.

Graham, H. (1993) *Hardship and Health in Women's Lives*. Brighton: Harvester Wheatsheaf.

Graham, M. (1997) 'Food allocation in rural Peruvian households: concepts and behaviour regarding children', *Social Science and Medicine*, **44**(1): 1697–709.

Haddad, L. (ed.) (1992) *Understanding how Resources are Allocated within Households*, IFPRI Policy Brief No 8.

Haddad, L., Pena, C. and Slack, A. (1994) *Poverty and Nutrition within Households: Review and New Evidence*, IFPRI in collaboration with WHO, March.

Heise, L., Pitanguy, J. and German, A. (1994) *Violence Against Women: The Hidden Health Burden*. Washington DC: World Bank.

Hyndman, S. (1990) 'Housing, damp and health among British Bengalis in East London', *Social Science and Medicine*, **30**(1): 131–41.

Kettel, B. (1996) 'Women, health and the environment', *Social Science and Medicine*, **42**(10): 1367–80.

Malik, I., Bukhtiari, N., Good, M.J., Iqbal, M., Azim, S., Nawaz, M. and Ashraf, L. (1992) 'Mothers' fear of child death: a study in urban and rural communities in Northern Punjab, Pakistan', *Social Science and Medicine*, **35**: 1043–53.

Manderson, L., Jenkins, J. and Tanner, M. (1993) 'Women and tropical diseases: introduction', *Social Science and Medicine*, **37**(4): 441–3.

McCarthy, P. (1985) 'Respiratory conditions: effects of housing and other factors', *Journal of Epidemiology and Community Health*, **39**(1): 15–19.

Messer, E. (1997) 'Intra-household allocation of food and healthcare: current findings and understandings – introduction', *Social Science and Medicine*, **44**(11): 1675–84.

Michelson, E. (1993) 'Adam's rib awry? women and schistosomiasis', *Social Science and Medicine*, **37**(4): 493.

Miles, A. (1988) *Women and Mental Illness: The Social Context of Female Neurosis*. Brighton: Harvester Wheatsheaf.

Miller, B. (1997) 'Social class, gender and household food allocations to children in South Asia', *Social Science and Medicine*, **44**(11): 1685–95.

Norboo, T., Yahya, M., Bruce, N., Heady, J. and Ball, K. (1991) 'Domestic pollution and respiratory illness in a Himalayan village', *International Journal of Epidemiology*, **20**(3): 749–57.

Oakley, A. (1974) *The Sociology of Housework*. London: Martin Robertson.

Oakley, A. (1976) *Housewife*. Harmondsworth: Penguin.

Plichta, S. (1992) 'The effects of woman abuse on health care utilisation and health status', *Women's Health, Jacobs Institute*, **2**(3): 154–62.

Rathgeber, E. and Vlassoff, C. (1993) 'Gender and tropical disease: a new research focus', *Social Science and Medicine*, **37**(4): 513–20.

Reuben, R. (1993) 'Women and malaria: special risks and appropriate control strategy', *Social Science and Medicine*, **37**(4): 473–80.

Rodda, A. (1991) *Women and the Environment*. London: Zed Press.

Rogers, B. and Schlossman, N. (eds) (1990) *Intra-household Resource Allocation*. Tokyo: UN University Press.

Romito, P. (1990) 'Postpartum depression and the experience of motherhood', *Acta Obstetricia & Gynaecologica Scandinavia*, **69** (supplement 154): 1–37.

Rosenberg, H. (1984) 'The home is the workplace: hazards, stress and pollutants in the household' in W. Chaukin (ed.) *Double Exposure: Women's Hazards on the Job and at Home*. New York: Monthly Review.

Sen, A. (1990) 'More than 100 million women are missing', *New York Review of Books*, 20 December: 61–6.

Sims, J. (1994) *Women, Health and Environment: An Anthology*. Geneva: WHO.

Stark, E. and Flitcraft, A. (1991) 'Spouse abuse' in M. Rosenberg and M. Fenley (eds) *Violence in America: A Public Health Approach*. Oxford: Oxford University Press.

United Nations (1991) *The World's Women 1970–1990: Trends and Statistics*, Social Statistics and Indicators, Series K. no 8, New York.

United Nations Development Programme (1995) *Human Development Report 1995*.

Vlassoff, C. and Bonilla, E. (1994) 'Gender related differences in the impact of tropical diseases on women: what do we know?', *Biosocial Sciences*, **26**: 37–53.

World Bank (1993) *World Development Report 1993: Investing in Health*. Oxford: Oxford University Press.

2 PAID AND UNPAID WORK IN MENTAL HEALTH: TOWARDS A NEW PERSPECTIVE

Sarah Payne

Following on from the previous analysis of domestic work in a range of settings, this chapter highlights the links between paid and unpaid work in relation to occupational health problems. In recent years researchers have begun to pay increasing attention to the influence of both work and unemployment on mental health. However, many questions are still unanswered and the implications of these issues for occupational health provision remain largely unexplored. This chapter creates a framework for moving the debate on. It explores the different dimensions of work that can affect mental health in either positive or negative ways. Characteristics such as security, control, isolation and levels of social support in both paid and unpaid work can all influence mental wellbeing but these traits are not equally distributed between different types of work. As a result, gender, class and race inequalities in mental health can often be reinforced by subjective experiences of work and unemployment.

Introduction

Mental health problems in the workplace are an internationally recognised problem (WHO, 1978, cited in Waldegrave, 1991, 1985; Karasek and Theorell, 1990). One of the aims of the World Health Organisation's 'Health for All' programme was that people 'should be effectively protected against work-related health risks' (WHO, 1978, cited in Waldegrave, 1991, p. xi). Britain is no exception to the phenomenon of increasing rates of mental ill health found among working populations. The recent British Psychiatric Morbidity surveys estimate that one in seven people in the general population is suffering from some level of psychiatric disorder (Meltzer et al., 1995). Another study suggested that around 6 or 7 million people in Britain are suffering from some form of mental health disorder at any one time (Thompson, 1994).

While these are measures of mental ill health based on clinical definitions of psychiatric symptoms, self-reported measures of mental distress show similarly high levels (Payne, 1991). Many of these people are in paid work, and will spend up to a third of their day in a place of employment (Jenkins, 1991; Nichol and Bacon, 1991). Mental illness is a major reason for lost working days in Britain, with an estimated 70–80 million days lost each year, at an annual cost of over £3700 million (Waldegrave, 1991; Thompson, 1994). Promoting the mental health of people in paid employment formed part of the Conservative government's 'Health of the Nation' strategy to improve the health of the British population by the year 2000 (Miller, 1991; DOH, 1992). While this goal was not achieved by the target date of 1995, mental health in the workplace has been more widely studied and discussed in Britain in recent years, as it has in other countries (Jenkins and Coney, 1991; Floyd et al., 1994).

At the macro-level the association between mental wellbeing and paid work has been studied through an examination of the relationship between economic trends and patterns of ill health (see Brenner, 1973; Eyer, 1984, for example). At the micro-level, research has explored ways in which paid employment may affect mental health, both positively, in the opportunities it offers for improved mental wellbeing, and negatively, through the stress it provokes, either in itself or when it is in conflict with other responsibilities (Jahoda, 1982; Warr, 1987; Jenkins, 1991). The economic impact of mental illness at work, in particular the effect of poor mental health on individual work performance and on sickness absences and labour turnover has also been an area of concern (Jenkins, 1991; Miller, 1991). Finally, there has been a growing interest in the development of occupational mental health strategies, particularly employment-based counselling to improve output and morale (Lisle, 1994; Coldwell and Brayley, 1996).

Thus, while occupational health literature has traditionally focused on the physical health of employees, there is an increasing interest in 'proactive' strategies for promoting mental wellbeing in the workplace (see, for example, Nichol and Bacon, 1991; Lisle, 1994; Spiers, 1996).

Debate continues about the ways in which work might be restructured to reduce negative influences on mental wellbeing (Karasek and Theorell, 1990; Miller, 1991; Nichol and Bacon, 1991).

This growing focus on mental health at work is happening at a time when the labour market and the organisation of employment are changing on a global scale (Townsend, 1993). Such changes have affected not only where and how paid work is carried out, but also the security of employment, and the kind of working conditions employees might experience. These are all factors which can have a particular impact on the mental health of workers. It is likely, therefore, that psychosocial wellbeing will become increasingly central to our understanding of the nature of the relationship between paid employment and health (Lisle, 1994).

To some extent this shift reflects labour conditions in rich countries rather than those experienced in developing countries and in 'free trade zones' where physical health hazards continue to present a major impediment to health (Taylor, 1985; LaBotz, 1994; Doyal, 1995). However, the international nature of social polarisation in labour markets means that some workers in the developed world may increasingly find that they have more in common with workers in less developed countries than with the more affluent in their own country. Similarly, despite the continuing threat to physical health of appalling work conditions across the globe, hazards to mental health and the psychosocial aspects of work are as important to workers in a Mexican *maquiladora* as they are to workers in a British insurance company. Pervasive sexual harassment, fears about job security and concern over the safety of children in the absence of childcare add mental health stresses to the physical hazards presented by industrial pollution, chemical exposure and poor workplace design (LaBotz, 1994).

While paid work is a real source of income, it also has a wider meaning. The notion of 'paid work' as an activity is quite different from that of 'unpaid work', with greater value and esteem being given to what is seen as real 'work'. Yet for the individual worker (especially those who are female) there is often an overlap between these roles and responsibilities, with a complex relationship between different parts of their lives. Thus, to understand the ways in which paid work influences mental health we need to move away from a traditional focus on 'work' as paid employment in the external workplace, towards an understanding of the range of circumstances and conditions in which different kinds of labour are carried out:

In the future, it may become increasingly difficult and undesirable to separate work/home or work/family domains in either industrialised or developing countries. As the trend towards smaller workplaces takes hold, for
example, a related increase may occur in the number of people who work
from within their homes (particularly in the burgeoning service sector).
(World Health Organisation, 1993, p. 2)

Feminist research has highlighted the inadequacy of a focus on paid
employment alone which follows 'the traditional but artificial distinction between paid and unpaid work' (Hunt and Annandale, 1993;
Popay *et al.*, 1993). The health impact of both paid employment and
domestic labour is interrelated with other factors, and research needs
to reflect the different sources of stress and wellbeing in people's lives,
through:

A reconceptualisation of labour conditions to take account of women's
unpaid work, of the possible interactions between formal and domestic
labour in women's lives; and of both the material and the psychological
aspects of labour conditions. (Popay *et al.*, 1993, p. 31)

This perspective has been used increasingly to explore women's
working lives. It now needs to be extended to both sexes since there is
also a lack of research on the ways in which men's family roles
combine with paid work to affect health chances (Arber and Lahelma,
1993). To take this approach further requires a model that incorporates a number of different factors affecting the relationship between
'work' and mental wellbeing, factors that have usually been treated
separately by researchers.

The impact of occupational hazards on mental health has been
considered mainly by health psychologists. This has been done with
little reference to the literature either on unemployment and mental
health (Peterson, 1994) or on domestic work. These psychological
studies have focused on factors such as locus of control, job satisfaction
and opportunities for self-esteem, but few have connected the impact of
these on the individual's circumstances away from their paid work.

Some writers, such as Peterson (1994), have taken this further,
arguing that questions of control and autonomy only make sense if
considered alongside the broader sociopolitical dimensions of employment. However, there has been little attempt to extend this into the
interrelationship between work and the domestic sphere. While some
studies have explored the impact on physical and mental health of
carrying a number of roles in combination – for example, being a paid
worker, a houseworker, and a parent (Hunt and Annandale, 1993;
Popay *et al.*, 1993) – these findings have not been incorporated into
more traditional occupational health research.

There are also a number of problems with the literature on unemployment and mental health. Many studies have focused on unemployment as a negative factor without questioning the content and health consequences of the job which has been lost. Within such models, all unemployment is viewed as equally negative – and again the complexities of compensating factors are lost. Recent analysis of the impact of unemployment on health has begun to consider why some people are less affected than others, using a broader model of effects (Bartley, 1994; Hammarstrom, 1994). Such an approach, which reflects the way health-related factors can cross categories and accumulate, needs now to be extended to the analysis of paid work. For example, a lack of control over workplace decisions may be offset by control in other spheres of activity, and vice versa (Lennon and Rosenfield, 1992; Hammarstrom, 1994).

The rest of this chapter sets out some of the themes which might be included in an alternative model of work and mental health, based on labour and labour conditions in both paid and unpaid employment. The focus is primarily on evidence relating to mental health effects of paid and unpaid work in developed countries, but the argument – that we can only understand the relationship between work and mental health when we take account of the complexity of different kinds of labour – is a more general one that can be applied across all societies. The final section returns to the implications of such a model for the occupational health services. We begin with a brief review of how mental health has been associated with employment status.

Conceptualising the mental health impact of work

Paid employment appears to be a significant protective factor for mental health for both men and women. Most research shows poorer mental health among the unemployed, and some also shows higher rates of suicide and parasuicide (Crombie, 1989; Platt and Robinson, 1991; Lahelma, 1992; Platt, 1992; Gunnell et al., 1995). A major study of working-class women in London found that paid employment was one of four factors which appeared to protect them against depression in the face of adverse life events (Brown and Harris, 1978). Other studies have similarly found paid employment to be a protective factor in women's mental health (Arber and Lahelma, 1993; Bromberger and Matthews, 1994; Glass and Fujimoto, 1994). Marriage seems to exert a negative effect on women's mental health, compared with a positive effect for men (Radloff, 1980), and one reason for this may be the way in which marriage and parenthood limit women's opportunities for paid employment.

However, these data are difficult to interpret since there is also a so-called 'healthy worker' effect. This reflects the fact that in times of recession and labour surplus it is the mentally unhealthy who are most likely to lose their job, both because of poorer work records, including sickness absences, and also because they are more likely to have been recently recruited, or work on part-time or short-term contracts, and are therefore more easily removed from paid employment (Hawton et al., 1988). Moreover, while unemployment status itself appears to have negative effects on wellbeing, leaving a distressing and stressful work situation can have a positive effect on mental health (Graetz, 1993; Buck, 1997). Clearly any association between unemployment and mental health is therefore likely to be complex, affected by factors such as the length of unemployment, how desirable the job was, the social disadvantage experienced as a result of unemployment, and the effect of unemployment on social relationships (Warr, 1987).

Research findings relating to women as a separate group are especially difficult to interpret. While women who are full-time housewives appear to have poorer health prospects than those in paid work, women who are in full-time employment in manual occupations and lower non-manual occupations suffer adverse health consequences more often than those in professional and managerial jobs (Arber, 1991). Women in well paid employment can more easily afford to pay for childcare and domestic services, and are also more likely to have flexibility over the timing of their paid work reducing the negative effects of having to carry a number of different responsibilities (Arber et al., 1985; Arber, 1991; Popay et al., 1993). Thus part-time, low paid employment may offer women the worst prospects for mental wellbeing.

Here again, however, there is the possibility of a 'healthy worker' effect, since women who have both paid work and domestic responsibilities may be those with better mental health (Martikainen, 1995), while those suffering from depression and anxiety may be less able to take on additional roles (Arber et al., 1985) or may be advised by their medical practitioner to give up paid work (Roberts, 1985).

This suggests that those aspects of paid employment which offer a protective effect are both complicated and interwoven with circumstances beyond paid work. Over 50 years ago Jahoda suggested that in addition to the financial benefits of employment, paid work offers other, latent benefits: giving a time structure to the day; offering opportunities for shared experiences, which are linked to common rather than individual goals; personal status; and opportunities or reasons to engage in physical activity (Jahoda, 1942, cited in Bartley, 1994). Warr (1982) summarised the benefits of employment as being 'the provision of money, activity, variety, temporal structure, social contacts, and a status and identity within society's institutions and networks' (Warr, 1982, p. 7). In these accounts, having paid employment offers a number of intricate and interrelated health benefits, over and above the financial reward.

What then of unpaid employment and mental health? Housework has often been described in terms of the negative effect it has on mental health – the low status which the position occupies, combined with the never-ending nature of the work itself, the lack of clarity over the role, the lack of structure, and the fragmentation (Gove and Tudor, 1973; Oakley, 1974; see also Doyal, this volume). Domestic labour is largely carried out in isolation from others, and although childcare may offer opportunities for socialising with those in the same situation, having children at home may also make the housework more difficult to complete (Oakley, 1974).

Those responsible for both domestic work and paid employment may suffer the negative effects of housework combined with the additional stress of a paid job – and particularly the difficulty of combining these roles in ways that satisfy others as well as themselves. It is no coincidence that women whose partners support their paid employment to the point of sharing the domestic labour are less at risk of both mental and physical ill health than those who carry the burden alone (Arber et al., 1985). When returning to the labour market after having children, the paid work women take on is often at a lower level of skill and remuneration (Arber and Lahelma, 1993), and with less security, than earlier employment (Payne, 1991). It appears paradoxical that this paid employment tends to improve mental health. Yet not all women benefit to the same extent, illustrating the need for a more complex approach to understanding these issues.

As we have seen, the category 'not in paid employment', is a heterogeneous one, with different implications dependent on what is offered or seen as the reason for being outside the labour market. Retirement and childcare are located in a different plane to sickness and disability, which are in a different plane again to being unable to find a job. Yet all exist as 'other' in the context of paid work. Such categories are not static over time or place, but they are nonetheless powerful with an impact at the individual level – being 'just a housewife', for example.

What is needed, therefore, is a recognition in occupational health strategies of such complexities. The woman who goes back to paid work in a less skilled job and who still retains the major responsibility for housework may enjoy improved mental health for a range of reasons – a change of environment, the structure the work imposes, increased opportunities for social contact, and the status which attaches to paid employment but not to the housewife role. These positive effects may exist even when the job allows little opportunity for self-determination, when the working conditions are poor, when it replicates the kind of emotional demands made on the woman at home or when the combination of paid work and domestic labour is exhausting.

Similarly, being 'just' a mother and housewife does not automatically lead to depression. What is it that allows some women to take on this role and enjoy good mental health? Again, there are a number of interlinked aspects: the work itself may be enjoyable and rewarding, it may offer sufficient opportunities for social contact where the woman is involved with a network of other carers, and for some women the conditions in which the work is carried out may be such that it is less stressful. Having access to a car, for example, allows more opportunities for social contact.

If we reconceptualise work or labour, then, as comprising a range of components, each of which is represented in different combinations in particular kinds of activity, we can draw closer to what it is about these activities and their interaction with each other that affects mental wellbeing. We can then consider how far these factors are present or absent in different contexts and determine whether their effects are positive or negative. This is particularly relevant as the traditional boundaries between paid work and unpaid work, the public sphere of employment and the private domestic world, are breaking down.

Control and autonomy

One characteristic of paid work that is related to mental health is the degree of control the worker has over her own labour – the way in which the work is carried out, the pace of the work, and relationships with fellow workers, for example (Lisle, 1994). Warr (1982) described this as 'decision latitude' – how far decisions can be made by the individual rather than by others.

Modern inflexible systems of production – where tasks have been broken down into small components and individual workers have very little control over their own work (either the speed at which they would work or the nature of the task itself) – have been widely criticised (Jahoda, 1982; Karasek and Theorell, 1990; Carayon, 1994). Studies show increased stress in situations where the worker is unable to control the pace of work, and where the lack of decision latitude creates a passivity at work and increases job strain (Peterson, 1994; Doyal, 1995; Stansfeld et al., 1997). In this situation workers are particularly at risk of anxiety, depression, apathy, low self-esteem and low self-confidence (Warr, 1991). A study of pregnant female employees with low job control found they suffered increased symptoms of stress, and were more likely to deliver pre-term babies and babies with low birthweight for gestational age (Henriksen et al., 1994).

In the UK, the Whitehall study of civil servants reported that low job control was associated with an increased risk of coronary heart disease (Marmot, 1996; Stansfeld et al., 1997). One element of this is the possible impact of low control within the broader social and political context: high levels of unemployment in a particular industry, for example, may increase the adverse effects of managerial control, by reducing opportunities to move to another workplace (Peterson, 1994). This has remained relatively unexplored, although Doyal highlights such complexities in the context of the experience of sexual harassment at work:

> The woman who is harassed at work is in a classically stressful situation. She does not want this interference in her life but equally she may not want to risk her job. Thus her only choice is to remain in a constant state of vigilance, and research has shown that a chronic stress response of this kind can lead to long-term physical problems such as high blood pressure, ulcers or heart disease. In addition, mental health problems may well result from the need to deny fear suppress anger and cope with the irrational guilt that so many harassed women feel. (Doyal, 1995, p. 168)

In unpaid labour, while some aspects of childcare could be seen as relatively autonomous, there are elements of childcare, and other kinds of unpaid caring work (such as care for older dependants) and also elements of domestic labour where autonomy is restricted. Women who are full-time housewives often have less autonomy than those in paid employment, and this is particularly true of financial autonomy (Arber and Lahelma, 1993; Doyal, 1995). Peterson's (1994) argument that the effect of workplace control needs to be considered within the wider sociopolitical environment is also relevant to domestic labour. Partners can exert control over working conditions by taking charge of finances and by demanding the creation of a particular type of domestic environment (Land, 1983; Wilson, 1987). Graham's research on women's poverty found that newly separated and divorced women often felt better off than before, despite being poorer, because they were free to spend their income in a different way (Graham, 1987). The threat of 'unemployment' may also affect women in the home, and the extent to which they feel in control of their own work. One study suggested that where women do have an element of control over their paid work this can moderate the negative effects on mental wellbeing of demands made by the family (Lennon and Rosenfield, 1992).

Security and insecurity

Lack of paid work can adversely affect mental health, although this effect is mediated by factors such as the presence or absence of social support, and the experience of isolation and loneliness, as well as the length of time the unemployment lasts and the extent to which it is associated with social disadvantage. Insecurity within paid employment also exerts a toll on mental health. One aspect of the restructuring of the labour market has been to increase job insecurity among parts of the workforce. More people are now working on short-term contracts or in part-time work with no job security, and this can increase stress-related symptoms and damage mental health in particular (Carayon, 1994; Hammarstrom, 1994; Lisle, 1994). However, the effect of this is not evenly distributed. Racist and discriminatory employment practices mean that unemployment is more common among people in the lower occupational groups, and among people from minority ethnic groups (Dex, 1982; Newnham, 1986). The higher levels of treatment for mental ill health among some groups, in particular people from Afro-Caribbean origins, may in part be the result of this mixture of higher unemployment and lower job security (Knowles, 1991).

Labour-related stress may also be caused by absence of feedback concerning performance at work, with higher levels of stress found among those employees without good levels of supervision (Warr, 1991). Similarly, one of the adverse effects of domestic labour identified by Gove and Tudor (1973) is that it is often performed without comment from others. One of the housewives in Oakley's classic study of housework said that the worst thing about being a housewife was, 'being taken for granted':

He never says anything about the way I keep the flat. If I say that to him he says it always looks nice. Housework is a waste of time really. (Oakley, 1974, p. 113)

Isolation and social contact

One of the major reasons offered for the protective effect of paid employment on mental health is the way in which paid work creates opportunities to reduce isolation and increase social contact (Jahoda, 1982; Warr, 1982). Studies of depression among women with caring and domestic responsibilities suggest one of the reasons paid work is valued is that it offers the opportunity to get out of the house and develop relationships with others (Brown and Harris, 1978; Houston et al., 1992). Having good social support is also a major factor in decreasing the risk of depression and anxiety (Brown and Harris, 1978, 1989). Studies of unemployed people have found that those who have high levels of social activity appear to have better mental health, and fewer psychological symptoms, than those with low levels of social activity (Wilson and Walker, 1993; Bartley, 1994; Hammarstrom, 1994). Unemployed people who report feelings of loneliness are more likely to have poorer mental health than those who do not (Leeflang et al., 1992).

Social support and social contact, however, have to be seen in conjunction with other factors. The support gained through paid work does appear to reduce some of the other, less positive, effects of paid work and the stress of having additional external duties such as domestic responsibilities and childcare (Stansfeld et al., 1997), while social support may be less able to moderate stress among women who are not in paid employment outside the home (Houston et al., 1994). In fact, one of the reasons why women with a number of roles and responsibilities have better mental health than those who have wholly domestic and parental roles may be that women with multiple roles have greater opportunity for social integration (Arber and Lahelma, 1993).

While social support is usually beneficial, enforced social contact for example, in open-plan office spaces – can be damaging. Similarly, social support may operate better in a situation which confers a higher status – as in paid employment – than one which confers a low status, as in the case of housework. There may also be differences in the nature of the contact itself. Hunt and Annandale (1993) in their study of the influences of both paid and unpaid work on the health of men and women found that men were more likely than women to have close contacts and friends in their paid workplace. Social support in the workplace may offset low support at home (Stansfeld *et al.*, 1997), while support from the family may offset stress in paid employment (Makowska, 1995).

There is an increasing number of people who do their paid work at home, and are therefore unlikely to gain social support through this employment. If this involves computer technology, it can be used to connect the worker with others to reduce isolation. However, such benefits will not extend to all homeworkers. Where they are paid by results there may not be time for the homeworker to choose social interaction over paid activity. And a large proportion of workers in this category are low paid and employed in repetitive and monotonous tasks such as filling envelopes and making up cardboard boxes. Many of this group are women, whose childcare responsibilities keep them at home. Thus there is an increasing social polarisation in this sector of the labour market. Advantages such as on-line social support will not extend to all homeworkers, and some workers will remain extremely isolated, with consequent effects on their mental health.

Economic and other resources

The most obvious benefit from paid employment is financial, and the most obvious cost of not having paid work is the lack of regular income. This means reliance on another source of funding – usually the state benefits system or the earnings of another person. The amount received from paid work is associated with mental health both in terms of actual income, and what can be purchased with this, and what the income represents in terms of status. Self-esteem is linked with what the individual feels herself or himself to be worth and whether income reflects that worth. Thus payment which is inadequate on any of these measures may detract from mental wellbeing.

With the abolition of the Wages Councils which protected the lowest paid in Britain, together with high rates of unemployment and low levels of state benefit, more people are now living on an income which leaves them and those they are responsible for either in poverty or on the margins of it (Gordon and Pantazis, 1997). Some groups are more vulnerable to this than others – women, people in minority ethnic groups, and those in unskilled occupations are more likely to be on low pay, and are likely to benefit less from the positive effects of employment. Similarly, women returning to the labour market after caring for children are likely to return to a lower occupational level than before (Land, 1983; Payne, 1991) and this too may have negative effects on the opportunities for mental health through the financial reward. This needs to be offset against the positive effect of having money of one's own for those women who have previously been totally reliant on the earnings of another (Glendinning and Millar, 1992; Doyal, 1995).

Obviously unpaid work cannot offer the advantages that are obtained from the receipt of an income. While those responsible for housework and childcare may receive money from a partner, this is paid not as a wage but as an 'allowance', as an intra-household transfer, and women have no legal right to this within marriage. Money which is received through the state benefit system is similarly not a wage but an allowance and neither form of payment represents a boost to self-esteem in the way that an income from paid work does. The universal child benefit, paid in Britain to the person responsible for children, most of whom are women, is however a significant source of independent money despite the low rate at which it is paid and has been vigorously defended by groups such as the Child Poverty Action Group and by the women's movement in Britain whenever it has been threatened (Pascall, 1997).

Opportunities for satisfaction and self-esteem

Paid work and occupational status remain the most important sources of social status in society, and to that extent paid work offers an important source of individual self-esteem (Jahoda, 1942, cited in Bartley, 1994; Warr, 1982). Work which has a low social value increases stress and decreases mental wellbeing, as does work which gives those performing it little opportunity to gain satisfaction from using their skills (Warr, 1991). One of the reasons for the poorer mental health and higher rates of depression among women engaged full time in domestic labour is the low status such work has in western society (Oakley, 1974; Doyal, 1995 and this volume).

For most 'houseworkers', the task of domestic labour is combined with childcare, which may offer more intrinsic status and more opportunities for satisfaction, although childcare itself is also a potential source of stress (Oakley, 1974; Romito, 1994). Women who are both mothers and in paid employment in higher status occupations have the best health of all. While some of this may be due to the more flexible nature of the work (Arber *et al.*, 1985; Arber, 1991) and the greater ease with which paid work can be combined with domestic responsibilities (including the ability to pay someone else to do some of it), it also appears to come from the status of the work itself (Romito, 1994).

Housework may also offer little opportunity for inherent job satisfaction. Housework is generally undone very quickly and one of its key features is the need to replicate the work continuously (Gove and Tudor, 1973; Oakley, 1974). The advent of labour-saving devices does not reduce this need for repetition of the same task, but reduces the time spent in the task and the use of specialist skills. This low level of satisfaction from housework is an important part of the explanation for the lower levels of self-esteem among housewives compared with women in paid employment (Romito, 1994). Warr (1991) suggests that the low level of demands made on a paid worker, in terms of skills needed, combined with an absence of task variety, are significant factors reducing the opportunity to feel a sense of achievement in one's work and thus leading to greater stress and lower self-esteem, and this can clearly be extended also to unpaid domestic work.

Sexual harassment in paid work also affects self-esteem and health, producing anxiety, depression, anger, guilt and fear, as well as sleeplessness, sexual and eating problems and other physical symptoms (LaBotz, 1994; Doyal, 1995). Similarly, in the private sphere, harassment, abuse and violence all damage women's self-esteem and mental wellbeing, as well as constituting a threat to physical health (Doyal, 1995).

Conclusion: mental health and occupational health services

This chapter has suggested that to analyse the impact of work on mental health we need a model which is able to incorporate the variety of people's lives – including the other areas of 'work' they may be responsible for and the range of ways in which these factors interact. Issues such as control and autonomy cannot be understood merely in the context of paid work, since they may also be influenced by factors outside paid work. It is the interaction between these settings that helps to construct opportunities for mental health. Similarly, social contact and isolation may be more or less important to the individual, depending on their experience of social support elsewhere.

This model may seem to suggest that there are limits to what occupational health services can achieve, since so many of the factors affecting mental wellbeing are external to the paid workplace. However, as the World Health Organisation has argued, while a distinction can be made between 'work-related' and 'work-caused' mental health problems, this distinction does not diminish the responsibility of employers to provide safe working environments. Neither does it diminish the responsibility of society to regulate workplaces (WHO, 1985). In a recent British High Court decision on a claim for damages for an employment-related injury to mental health, the judge ruled that 'an employer owes a duty to his [sic] employees not to cause them psychiatric damage by the volume or character of the work they are required to perform' (Burrell, 1997, p. 3).

An appreciation of this interaction between work in paid employment and work elsewhere is invaluable in devising intervention in paid work. Thus occupational health services may not be able to increase the social support workers gain when away from their workplace. However, recognising the way in which paid work increases or limits opportunities for support at work helps to identify interventions to maximise opportunities for such support in the workplace. It also encourages a consideration of the ways in which services such as counselling may have indirect consequences for social support away from paid work, which in turn may affect workplace performance.

Similarly, a recognition of the mental health consequences of harassment, bullying and abuse may lead to the creation of employment-based counselling services which then help people with these problems when they are employment related and also those which are not. How far occupational health services will in fact develop in such a direction depends in part on the extent to which such an approach is seen as cost effective in terms of economic measures of success – productivity and sickness-related absence, for example. However, occupational health as a discipline also needs to recognise this interconnectedness of factors impacting on mental health in order to target strategies appropriately.

References

Arber, S. (1991) 'Revealing women's health' in H. Roberts (ed.) *Women's Health Counts*. London: Routledge.

Arber, S., Dale, A., and Gilbert, G.N. (1985) 'Paid employment and women's health: a benefit or source of role strain?', *Sociology of Health and Illness*, **7**(3): 375–400.

Arber, S. and Lahelma, E. (1993) 'Inequalities in women's and men's ill-health – Britain and Finland compared', *Social Science and Medicine*, **37**(8): 1055–68.

Bartley, M. (1994) 'Unemployment and ill health: understanding the relationship', *Journal of Epidemiology and Community Health*, **48**: 333–7.

Brenner, M.H. (1973) *Mental Illness and the Economy*. Boston: Harvard University Press.

Bromberger, J.T. and Matthews, K.A. (1994) 'Employment status and depressive symptoms in middle-aged women: a longitudinal investigation', *American Journal of Public Health*, **84**(2): 202–6.

Brown, G. and Harris, T. (1978) *The Social Origins of Depression*. London: Tavistock.

Brown, G.W. and Harris, T.O. (eds) (1989) *Life Events and Illness*. London: Unwin Hyman.

Buck, M. (1997) 'The price of poverty', *Critical Social Policy*, **17**(1): 79–97.

Burrell, I. (1997) 'How stress distorts a healthy view of life', *The Independent*, 13 June, p. 3.

Carayon, P. (1994) 'Stressful jobs and non-stressful jobs: a cluster analysis of office jobs', *Ergonomics*, **37**(2): 311–23.

Coldwell, B. and Brayley, K. (1996) 'Clinical psychology or counselling?', *Occupational Health*, July: 250–1.

Crombie, I.K. (1989) 'Trends in suicide and unemployment in Scotland, 1976–1986', *British Medical Journal*, **298**: 1180.

Crombie, I.K. (1990) 'Suicide in England and Wales and in Scotland: an examination of divergent trends', *British Journal of Psychiatry*, **157** (October): 529–32.

Darragh, P.M. (1991) 'Suicide among men in the highlands of Scotland', *British Medical Journal*, **302**: 1020.

Department of Health (1992) *The Health of the Nation: A Strategy for Health in England*. London: HMSO.

Dex, S. (1982) *Black and White School Leavers: the First Five Years of Work*. London: Department of Employment.

Doyal, L. (1995) *What Makes Women Sick? Gender and the Political Economy of Health*. Basingstoke: Macmillan.

Eyer, J. (1984) 'Capitalism, health and illness' in J. McKinlay (ed.) *Issues in the Political Economy of Health Care*. London: Tavistock.

Glass, J. and Fujimoto, T. (1994) 'Housework, paid work and depression among husbands and wives', *Journal of Health and Social Behaviour*, **35**(2): 179–91.

Glendinning, C. and Millar, J. (eds) (1992) *Women and Poverty in Britain in the 1990s*. Hemel Hempstead: Harvester Wheatsheaf.

Gordon, D. and Pantazis, C. (eds) (1997) *Breadline Britain*. Aldershot: Avebury.

Gove, W.R. and Tudor, J.F. (1973) 'Adult sex roles and mental illness', *American Journal of Sociology*, **78**: 813–35.

Graetz, B. (1993) 'Health consequences of employment and unemployment: longitudinal evidence for young men and women', *Social Science and Medicine*, **36**(6): 715–24.

Graham, H. (1987) 'Being poor: perceptions and coping strategies of lone mothers' in J. Brannen and G. Wilson (eds) *Give and Take in Families: Studies in Resource Distribution*. London: Allen & Unwin.

Gunnell, D., Peters, T., Kammerling, R. and Brooks, J. (1995) 'Relation between parasuicide, suicide, psychiatric admissions and socio-economic deprivation', *British Medical Journal*, **311**: 226–30.

Hammarstrom, A. (1994) 'Health consequences of youth unemployment review from a gender perspective', *Social Science and Medicine*, **38**(5): 699–709.

Hawton, K., Fagg, J. and Simkin, S. (1988) 'Female unemployment and attempted suicide', *British Journal of Psychiatry*, **152**: 632–7.

Henriksen, T.B., Hedegaard, M. and Secher, N.J. (1994) 'The relation between psychosocial job strain and preterm delivery and low birthweight for gestational age', *International Journal of Epidemiology*, **23**(4): 764–74.

Houston, B.K., Cates, D.S. and Kelly, K.E. (1992) 'Job stress, psychosocial strain, and physical health problems in women employed full-time outside the home and homemakers', *Women's Health*, **19**(1): 1–26.

Hunt, K. and Annandale, E. (1993) 'Just the job – is the relationship between health and domestic and paid work gender-specific?', *Sociology of Health and Illness*, **15**(5): 632–64.

Jahoda, M. (1982) *Employment and Unemployment: A Social-psychological Analysis*. Cambridge: Cambridge University Press.

Jenkins, R. (1991) 'Prevalence of mental illness in the workplace' in R. Jenkins and N. Coney (eds).

Jenkins, R. and Coney, N. (eds) (1991) *Prevention of Mental Ill Health at Work*. London: Department of Health/Confederation of British Industry.

Karasek, R. and Theorell, T. (1990) *Healthy Work, Stress, Productivity and the Reconstruction of Working Life*. New York: Basic Books.

Knowles, C. (1991) 'Afro-Caribbeans and schizophrenia: how does psychiatry deal with issues of race, culture and ethnicity?', *Journal of Social Policy*, **20**(2): 173–90.

LaBotz, D. (1994) 'Manufacturing poverty: the maquiladorization of Mexico', *International Journal of Health Services*, **24**(3): 403–8.

Lahelma, E. (1992) 'Unemployment and mental well-being: elaboration of the relationship', *International Journal of Health Services*, **22**(2): 261–74.

Land, H. (1983) 'Who still cares for the family?' in J. Lewis (ed.) *Women's Welfare, Women's Rights*. London: Croom Helm.

Leeflang, R.L., Klein-Hesselink, D.J. and Spruit, I.P. (1992) 'Health effects of unemployment – I Long-term unemployed men in a rural and an urban setting', *Social Science and Medicine*, **3**(4): 341–50.

Lennon, M.C. and Rosenfield, S. (1992) 'Women and mental health: the interaction of job and family conditions', *Journal of Health and Social Behaviour*, **33**(4): 316–27.

Lisle, J. (1994) 'Occupational health services' in M. Floyd, M. Povall and G. Watson (eds) *Mental Health at Work*. London: Jessica Kingsley.

Makowska, Z. (1995) 'Psychosocial characteristics of work and family as determinants of stress and wellbeing of women: a preliminary study', *International Journal of Occupational Medicine and Environmental Health*, **8**(3): 215–22.

Marmot, M.G. (1996) 'Socio-economic factors in cardiovascular disease', *Journal of Hypertension*, **14** (Suppl)(5): 201–5.

Martikainen, P. (1995) 'Women's employment, marriage, motherhood and mortality: a test of the multiple role and role accumulation hypotheses', *Social Science and Medicine*, **40**(2): 199–212.

Meltzer, H., Gill, B., Pettigrew, M. and Hinds, K. (1995) *The Prevalence of Psychiatric Morbidity among Adults Living in Private Households.* OPCS Surveys of Psychiatric Morbidity in Great Britain, Report 1. London: OPCS.

Miller, D. (1991) 'Work problems caused by mental ill health and their management' in R. Jenkins and N. Coney (eds).

Newnham, A. (1986) *Employment, Unemployment and Black People.* London: Runneymede Trust.

Nichol, D.K. and Bacon, A.D. (1991) 'Managing mental health problems for a large workforce' in R. Jenkins and N. Coney (eds).

Oakley, A. (1974) *Housewife.* London: Allen Lane.

Pascall, G. (1997) *Social Policy: A Feminist Analysis.* London: Routledge.

Payne, S. (1991) *Women, Health and Poverty: An Introduction.* Hemel Hempstead: Harvester Wheatsheaf.

Peterson, C.L. (1994) 'Work factors and stress: a critical review', *International Journal of Health Services,* **24**(3): 495–519.

Platt, S. (1986) 'Parasuicide and unemployment', *British Journal of Psychiatry,* **149**: 401–5.

Platt, S. (1992) 'Epidemiology of suicide and parasuicide', *Journal of Psychopharmacology,* **6** (2 Supplement): 291–9.

Platt, S. and Robinson, A. (1991) 'Parasuicide and alcohol: a 20 year survey of admissions to a regional poisoning treatment centre', *International Journal of Social Psychiatry,* **37**(3): 159–72.

Popay, J., Bartley, M. and Owen, C. (1993) 'Gender inequalities in health – social position, affective-disorders and minor physical morbidity', *Social Science and Medicine,* **36**(1): 21–32.

Radloff, L. (1980) 'Risk factors for depression: what do we learn from them?' in M. Guttentag (ed.) *The Mental Health of Women.* New York: Academic Press.

Renvoize, E. and Clyden, D. (1989) 'Correspondence: suicide and unemployment', *British Medical Journal,* **298**: 1180.

Roberts, H. (1985) *The Patient Patients.* London: Pandora.

Romito, P. (1994) 'Work and health in mothers of young children', *International Journal of Health Services,* **24**(4): 607–28.

Spiers, C. (1996) 'Suicide in the workplace', *Occupational Health* (July): 247–9.

Stansfeld, S.A., Rael, E.G.S., Head, J., Shipley, M. and Marmot, M.G. (1997) 'Social support and psychiatric sickness absence: a prospective study of British civil servants', *Psychological Medicine,* **27**(1): 35–48.

Taylor, D. (1985) 'Women: an analysis' in *Women: A World Report.* London: Methuen.

Thompson, D. (1994) 'Mental health and illness' in M. Floyd, M. Povall and G. Watson (eds) *Mental Health at Work.* London: Jessica Kingsley.

Townsend, P. (1993) *The International Analysis of Poverty.* Hemel Hempstead: Harvester Wheatsheaf.

Waldegrave, W. (1991) 'Introduction' in R. Jenkins and N. Coney (eds).

Warr, P.B. (1982) 'Psychological aspects of employment and unemployment', *Psychological Medicine,* **12**: 7–11.

Warr, P.B. (1987) *Work, Unemployment and Mental Health.* Oxford: Oxford University Press.

Warr, P.B. (1991) 'Job features and executive stress' in R. Jenkins and N. Coney, (eds).

Wilkinson, R. (1996) *Unhealthy Societies: The Afflictions of Inequality*. London: Routledge.

Wilson, G. (1987) 'Money: patterns of responsibility and irresponsibility in marriage' in J. Lewis (ed.) *Women's Welfare, Women's Rights*. London: Croom Helm.

Wilson, S.H. and Walker, G.M. (1993) 'Unemployment and health: a review', *Public Health*, **107**: 153–62.

World Health Organisation (1985) *Identification and Control of Work-related Diseases*. Technical Report No. 174. Geneva: WHO.

World Health Organisation (1993) *Health Promotion in the Workplace: Alcohol and Drug Abuse*. Technical Report No. 833. Geneva: WHO.

3 THE WELLBEING OF CARERS: AN OCCUPATIONAL HEALTH CONCERN

Liz Lloyd

As the previous chapter demonstrated, official concern about health and safety at work has traditionally been confined to hazards arising from paid employment. However, it is increasingly clear that the focus of policy makers and practitioners needs to be broadened to encompass a range of other labours that may not be defined as work but can certainly be damaging to health. This chapter argues that case with reference to the example of paid and unpaid caring. There is often very little difference between the hazards faced by those who are paid to care for others and those who do it for 'love', yet these carers are treated very differently in terms of the degree of protection afforded to their health. Policy changes are needed to minimise these inequalities but they will not be easy to achieve. Compromises may have to be struck, for example, between privacy and protection or between the rights of the carer and the needs and desires of the person being cared for.

Introduction

This chapter considers the health and wellbeing of carers, focusing on those who provide care for people in their own homes. Caring, both paid and unpaid, is examined as a form of work and the risks to carers, from the tasks they carry out and the environment within which they work, are considered. A central strand in the discussion is the similarity between paid and unpaid carers' experiences which shows not

54

only how knowledge of occupational hazards in paid employment can be applied to unpaid work but also how the division between paid and unpaid caring is increasingly breaking down. This suggests that occupational health knowledge is relevant to both spheres and that the parameters of occupational health research need to be expanded.

Conventional sociological theories of work have concentrated on paid employment, ignoring unpaid work (Tancred, 1995; Thomas, 1995; Rantalaiho, 1997). This has been challenged by feminist research on the hazards of domestic labour (Dennerstein, 1995; Doyal, 1995). However, little is known about the experiences and health status of care workers in domestic settings. This reflects a wider perception of caring as a 'natural', predominantly feminine role, which is outside the sphere of interest of work-related research.

The lack of knowledge about health issues associated with unpaid caring also reflects patterns of funding and support for occupational health research. This has generally concentrated on establishing simple cause and effect relationships between paid work and acute illnesses or accidents in preference to more exploratory research on the complex factors which contribute to workers' ill health (Daykin, 1990; Messing et al., 1993; Messing, 1994). The analysis in this chapter takes these broader issues into account as well as highlighting the direct effects of caring on health. First, it examines how the tasks of caring and the physical environment of the home affect carers' health and wellbeing. Second, it explores how the broader social and political contexts influence the ways in which caring is constructed, how carers experience their role and what this means for their health and wellbeing.

The activities of caring

The range of activities which can be included under the umbrella term 'caring' is vast. Parker and Lawton (1994) present a typology of tasks based on their analysis of the 1985 British General Household Survey data which provides a useful basis for this discussion. Clusters of tasks identified in this typology are: personal care, such as dressing, bathing and so on; physical help, such as help with walking, getting in and out of bed; practical help, such as paperwork, preparing meals or shopping; and other help, which includes taking out for visits.

The tasks identified by Parker and Lawton may also be undertaken by paid carers, although there is considerable variation between carers, whether paid or unpaid, in the range and combinations of tasks carried out and in the level of responsibility taken. Parker and Lawton

(1994) found that unpaid carers providing personal and physical help were most likely to be women, to care for longer hours, to be related to and to be co-resident with the cared-for person and to have sole or main responsibility for them. This group is sometimes referred to as being at the 'heavy end' of caring.

The tasks involved in caring work are, as Baldock and Ely (1996) point out, both complex and mundane. On the one hand, they include the mundane activities of 'washing, toileting, dressing, cooking, cleaning, eating, mobility and communication' (Baldock and Ely, 1996, p. 202) but, on the other hand, the way people conduct their ordinary lives reflects their individuality and identity, and this makes the support given to older and disabled people highly complex. Warren points out that the work of home helps cannot be understood solely in terms of the tasks performed but that it has 'personal significance' in terms of their relationships with the cared-for people (Warren, 1990, p. 71). An occupational health analysis, therefore, needs to take into account not only the tasks which are performed but also the nature of the roles and responsibilities of carers.

The hazards of caring

Analysis of the risks and hazards of caring reveals striking similarities between paid and unpaid spheres. First, the perception of both paid and unpaid caring as self-sacrificing vocations obscures occupational health problems. Nurses' reputation as 'angels' depends on their willingness to put up with difficult conditions. Carers can be caught in a similar bind, highly valued for their 'heroic' work but unable to demand better conditions for fear of being labelled self-seeking.

Second, both paid and unpaid caring can be emotionally demanding. Barnett and Marshall suggest that 'workers who have direct responsibility for the fate of others' are more likely to experience emotional stress than those who are responsible for inanimate objects (Barnett and Marshall, 1991, cited in Doyal, 1995, p. 166). Their stress is exacerbated when they are unable to provide a good standard of care because of inadequate resources.

The health effects of both paid and unpaid caring are influenced by shifts in social policy and the organisation of care. The current trend away from institutional and towards domiciliary settings has increased the amount of work carried out in people's own homes, with considerable implications for occupational health. For example, the pressure to maintain people in their own homes has not always taken into account the physical condition of their housing. Many older and disabled people are on low incomes and are therefore less likely to be able to maintain healthy and safe conditions either for living or working in. This affects the person cared for as well as the range of people who provide care and support.

However, unpaid care does differ in some respects from paid care. For example, many unpaid carers are over retirement age and the risks they face may be compounded by their own failing health. Second, unpaid carers have no legal protection as workers, although it should be remembered that protective legislation for paid workers is not always enforced, as discussed later in this chapter.

Research on the wellbeing of paid and unpaid carers identifies four main areas of concern: physical health, mental or emotional health, financial costs and stresses of combining paid employment and unpaid caring. Taking each of these in turn, the similarities and differences between the experiences of paid and unpaid carers are considered below.

Physical health

Research evidence on the physical health status of unpaid carers provides a mixed picture, with the differences being mainly to do with whether representative or non-representative research samples were used (Evandrou, 1996). Studies based on self-selected samples identify relatively high levels of illness and a strong perception among carers that caring has affected their health. Warner, for example, suggests that carers suffer from lasting tiredness, back problems, difficulty sleeping, depression, muscular pain, weepiness and frequent headaches (Warner, 1995, p. 23).

By the same token, Parker and Lawton's analysis of the British General Household Survey suggests that the effects of sex and age have become confounded with those of caring and that a causal relationship between caring and physical ill health is difficult to establish (Parker and Lawton, 1994). Hogman and Pearson (1995) make a similar point about the carers of people with schizophrenia, many of whom are the parents of the person cared for. Because many carers are above the average age of the population as a whole, it is difficult to disentangle the effects of age from those of caring.

Taylor *et al.* (1995) argue that research into the effects of caring on the physical health of carers has produced results which are suggestive rather than conclusive because there is a tendency to overlook significant variations in the responsibilities of carers. They agree with Parker (1992) that more emphasis should be placed on those at the 'heavy end' of caring. Hancock and Jarvis (1994) note that, in Britain, 11 per cent of carers spend more than 50 hours a week providing care and that the effects of caring on this group are more clearly evident than for carers in general. A similar point is made by Evandrou (1996). Using a multivariate analysis of the 1990 British General Household Survey, Evandrou concludes that 'caring for someone co-residentially, bearing the main responsibility on one's own, caring for someone with both physical and mental impairments and caring for over fifty hours a week are associated with less good health' (Evandrou, 1996, p. 226). The implication of this is that those carers who are at greatest risk should be targeted and prioritised by service providers.

However, there is a danger in this approach. In attempting to establish a sub-category of carers at greatest risk it overlooks the risks associated with particular tasks of caring. Carers who work long hours without breaks are undoubtedly at serious risk of poor health but some of the risks faced by both paid and unpaid carers are attached to what they do as a normal part of the caring routine, whether full time or part time. For example, all care workers, whatever their status, are at risk of back injury from lifting the people they care for. Evidence from occupational health research with paid health care staff, such as nurses, demonstrates that many physical health risks are relevant to all carers.

The occupational health of nurses has been relatively well researched and the lifting and handling of patients emerges as one of the riskiest tasks, clearly associated with back injuries. Back injuries are more common among nurses than among any other occupational group. It is estimated that, in Britain, 764,000 working days are lost annually through back problems in nurses (Fingret and Smith, 1995). Lunn and Waldron (1991) point out that 'in industry no-one would be expected to move weights in excess of ten stone without proper lifting gear, but this is an everyday occurrence on any adult ward' (Lunn and Waldron, 1991, p. 61).

Claims for compensation by injured staff have galvanised some British health trusts into action to reduce the risk of injury (National Audit Office, 1996). The introduction of hoists and other equipment to take the load is widely viewed as effective, although provision of these is inadequate and there is a widespread expectation that nurses will have to do the lifting unaided. Other preventive measures include the provision of height-adjustable beds, and sufficient space around beds and in toilets and bathrooms to enable nurses to manoeuvre themselves into appropriate positions to lift or assist patients. In addition, techniques in handling patients have been developed for staff, although research suggests that manual handling training has not had a significant impact on the levels of injuries (Ashton and Wright, 1995). Lunn and Waldron note that occupational health practitioners experience 'a feeling of profound frustration' at the continued high incidence of back problems in nurses despite research into its causes (Lunn and Waldron, 1991, p. 61).

How, then, does this evidence from studies of hospital-based nursing apply to the experiences of carers in domestic settings? Inadequate funding of community care means that it is increasingly difficult to make appropriate adaptations to ordinary family homes and to provide equipment which could reduce risk of back injury. In ordinary houses, especially where families live in overcrowded conditions, there is less likelihood that there will be adequate space to enable carers to manoeuvre themselves into positions to lift safely. Research by Twigg and Atkin (1994) reveals serious problems for both carers and the people cared for arising from the lengthy waiting lists for adaptations. One carer reported that she was told she would have to wait six months for bath aids which she requested after her husband became stuck in the bath (Twigg and Atkin, 1994, p. 63).

Many carers make their own provision and buy equipment privately but this exposes both the carer and the person they care for to the risk of being sold unsuitable or even unsafe equipment, especially in an unregulated, second-hand market. There are no systematic checks on the safety of equipment in domestic settings as there are in workplaces covered by legislation. In hospitals, the recommended practice is for two nurses to work together to lift patients, whereas carers in domestic settings often work alone and this increases the risk of back injury.

Skin problems, such as dermatitis are also strongly associated with nursing (National Audit Office, 1996) and with housework (Doyal, 1995). These result from exposure to toxic chemicals which are found in cleaning materials, disinfectants and chlorine bleaches and from wearing protective gloves. These substances are commonly used by carers, especially where they have responsibility for personal and physical care. While there may be regulations covering the use of particular substances in the workplace, these regulations do not necessarily extend into the home and neither do they take into account the cumulative effect of using such substances in more than one setting. As Doyal points out: 'toxic substances do not become safe simply because they cross the threshold of the home' (Doyal, 1995, p. 36).

Consideration of these two examples suggests a pressing need to acknowledge the hazards associated with both paid and unpaid caring. In addition, there is a need to conduct proper risk assessments in people's own homes, not only for the benefit of paid workers who visit these but also for those who both live and work in them.

Carers' mental and emotional health

The risks to carers' mental and emotional health have been examined relatively extensively (Chappell and Penning, 1996; Evandrou, 1996). Here, again, there are similarities between paid and unpaid caring. Hochschild's concept of 'emotional labour', which refers to the expectation that an individual worker will mask her true feelings and maintain a cheerful and positive exterior, can be readily applied to nurses (Hochschild, 1983; Smith, 1992). It is recognised that the sense of overload, the absence of support and lack of control over their work which many nurses experience can lead to poor mental health (Doyal, 1995).

However, the concept is also relevant to unpaid caring. A cheerful and good-natured disposition is generally regarded as crucial to the caring role. The gap which sometimes emerges between how carers feel internally and how they appear externally has significant consequences for their mental health. Unpaid carers, too, report feelings of exhaustion and depression arising from a sense of being overloaded and from being unsupported in their work.

The mental health risks of unpaid caring have been studied in their own right. Parker and Lawton argue that poor emotional health in unpaid carers can 'confidently be ascribed to caring' (Parker and Lawton, 1994, p. 23). Especially stressful is the work of caring for a relative with dementia (Chappell and Penning, 1996; Evandrou, 1996). Rising levels of dementia pose a challenge to policy makers throughout Europe and North America, since these will lead not only to more people requiring care but also more intensive care which is likely to create extra stress in carers (Salvage, 1995).

The conditions under which caring roles are taken on are an important aspect of stress in caring. Arber and Ginn (1995) note that co-residence between carers and disabled parents often begins at the onset or development of severe disability and that this is likely to be a cause of conflict and stress. Some carers report feelings of stress from what Twigg and Atkin (1994) refer to as 'restrictedness': that is, the way in which care giving constrains the carer. For example, where the person cared for has dementia, carers find it extremely difficult to take a break or even to go out to shop for basic essentials.

The high rates of suicide, alcoholism and drug abuse in the medical profession are cited as the effects of long hours and stressful work (BMA, 1992). Long hours of work are inevitably stressful in themselves, but the ability to exercise control over hours worked is also extremely important. Twigg and Atkin have developed the concept of the 'engulfment' mode of caring, which describes how the lives of some carers become completely subordinated to the lives of people cared for (Twigg and Atkin, 1994, p. 122). Being able to set limits on the extent of their caring responsibilities emerges as a central issue in Leat's research on carers in 'adult placement schemes' (Leat, 1990).

There are currently around 200 such schemes in Britain in which social services departments arrange for disabled adults and adults with learning difficulties or mental health problems to live with a family in which one member is paid as a carer (Hirst, 1996). Leat (1990) concludes from her research that co-resident paid carers often work beyond the limits of what they are employed to do, sometimes at personal and financial cost to themselves, and that they resent being taken for granted by the employing social services departments. What they perceived as important to their own health and wellbeing was the ability to exercise some control over the number of hours worked and to take reasonable breaks from work. These two points came up 'over and over again in interviews' (Leat, 1990, p. 33), demonstrating that these paid carers were able to perceive clearly the dangers of becoming 'engulfed' in their role.

Leat concludes that although non-resident paid carers often did unpaid overtime they were less resentful of this than those who were co-resident because they felt they had a degree of choice over their commitments and control over their time. Similarly, Salvage (1995) notes that establishing limits to caring and the ability to take breaks are key issues for unpaid carers. Drawing on evidence from eleven European countries she suggests that respite care is one of the most highly prized forms of support.

Leat (1990) also notes the significance of employment agencies for the non-resident paid carers. Agencies were able to look after the interests of carers, to negotiate on their behalf and to sort out any problems between carers and clients. This suggests that carers may need advocates in order to assert their views about the limits of their responsibilities.

Understanding stress in both paid and unpaid caring work requires careful consideration of the differences between carers, the nature of the caring relationship and the ways in which carers develop strategies for coping. Salvage argues that '"stress perceived" in matters of care is strongly shaped by what is seen as "justified" or normal by carers' (Salvage, 1995, p. 44). There are gender differences in carers' perceptions of their roles. Twigg and Atkin (1994) note that more women than men fell into the 'engulfment mode' and that more women found it difficult to establish autonomy and to recognise their own needs for support. They also identify strong moral overtones in the relationships between carers and professionals in health and social services. Their research showed how professionals drew heavily on their own personal values and assumptions in making judgements about carers and what they should or should not do. Such moral pressures make it extremely difficult for carers to assert their own needs.

Financial effects of caring

Caring is strongly associated with poverty, either because of dependence on benefits or because of poor wages. This is particularly so for long-term, unpaid carers. From a British perspective, Hancock and Jarvis note that 'people who had cared for more than ten years were financially disadvantaged in almost all respects compared with both non-carers and with people who had cared for shorter periods' (Hancock and Jarvis, 1994, p. 73). Similarly, Evandrou (1996) found that 26 per cent of all carers and 40 per cent of older carers were living in poverty. In Ireland, three quarters of unpaid carers have incomes at or below the level at which they felt 'financial strain as a result of caring' (McLaughlin, 1994, p. 282).

The link between poverty and ill health is well established and the higher levels of poverty experienced by carers suggests that carers are at increased risk of poor general health, as well as facing particular occupational hazards. The health problems experienced by carers are likely to persist over the long term, sometimes for some time after caring responsibilities have ceased.

Poverty also affects the physical environment of caring. Parker and Lawton (1994) note that, in Britain, unpaid carers with primary responsibility for personal and physical care (the 'heavy end' of caring) had lower rates of owner occupation than the general population and were significantly more likely to be living in overcrowded households (Parker and Lawton, 1994, p. 42). Housing problems are a particular issue for minority ethnic communities who are more likely to experience damp conditions, and to lack central heating and other household amenities (Atkin and Rollings, 1996).

The low incomes of paid care workers and many nurses can be similarly linked to the risk of poor health. The assumption that women's paid employment is an extension of their 'natural' caring role is often used as an excuse for their low wages. O'Donovan (1997) notes how Irish home helps are recruited by health boards on the understanding that they should be more interested in the opportunity to help others than in the level of pay they receive. In France, a system of tax allowances has encouraged families to employ unskilled paid workers to take on care work, facilitating carers' participation in paid work. This has, however, given rise to criticism about the pay and conditions of work of the care workers (Joel and Martin, 1994).

Paid employment and unpaid caring

Combining paid employment with unpaid caring responsibilities has both advantages and disadvantages for the physical and emotional health of carers. Paid employment is an important means of survival for both carer and the person cared for, particularly in poorer families. Evidence suggests that many carers are unable to work as much as they would like to (Hogman and Pearson, 1995; Caring Costs Alliance, 1996) and unpaid caring can, therefore, be seen to have 'opportunity costs'. Paid employment outside the home is also an opportunity for wider social contact for carers. Drawing on evidence from eleven European countries, Salvage (1995) argues that as well as providing an income, paid employment offers an opportunity for respite from caring and has a 'restorative' function.

Work helps to combat the isolation experienced by many carers and provides a sense of balance in their lives. Drew notes that combining paid employment with caring can 'bolster the caregiver's competence and offer more exposure to additional resources' (Drew, 1995, p. 327). In Nova Scotia, an evaluation of the Home Life Support Program, which provides payment to family members who give up paid employment to care for elderly relatives, found that full-time carers experienced higher levels of stress than those who combined caring responsibilities with work outside the home (Stryckman and Nahmiash, 1994).

However, many carers struggle to balance the demands of paid and unpaid work. Research in Britain by the Caring Costs Alliance (1996) shows that some employees feared that they would be sacked if their employers knew the extent of their caring responsibilities. Over a half of those interviewed said that they experienced higher levels of stress since having to combine paid work with caring responsibilities and 43 per cent were unsure about being able to continue in employment. These difficulties are rarely acknowledged in occupational health research.

From her research in Canada, Messing notes the frequency of stress among women workers and emphasises the need for occupational health specialists to 'include interactions with family responsibilities in their conceptions of workplace norms and standards' (Messing, 1994, p. 13). The occupational health of carers could therefore be improved by measures which accommodate the caring responsibilities of employees. Salvage argues that 'job sharing, paid care leave, flexible hours, the opportunity to make private telephone calls... could all help working carers to combine their two very important roles' (Salvage, 1995, p. 53).

Conditions of employment in Scandinavian countries include more rights to paid or unpaid leave for caring responsibilities and this has had a significant impact on women's participation in the paid workforce. Lingsom maintains that, in Norway, the feminist debate about the effect of caring on women's employment has largely subsided as 'caregiving is increasingly seen as a phase in an otherwise stable employment history for women' (Lingsom, 1994, p. 69).

Taken as a whole, this evidence suggests that a combination of paid work and unpaid caring can be beneficial to the health and wellbeing of carers but that conditions of employment need to be conducive to their caring roles in order to avoid stress.

The context of caring work

The discussion so far has concentrated on the direct effects of caring on health. The broader context of caring work is also significant for the development of an occupational health perspective.

The development of community care policies in industrial societies has coincided with global deregulation of labour markets and often stringent cuts in spending on welfare. The impact of these developments on both paid and unpaid carers is significant. Rigorous targeting of services to people with the greatest needs means that domiciliary care services are likely to be concentrated on people whose needs are complex but at the same time agencies strive to keep costs to a minimum. Unpaid carers are more likely, in times of financial stringency, to experience pressure to take on caring responsibilities but are less likely to be supported or to get respite care. What are the implications for the health and safety of care workers?

The financial constraints which exist in industrialised countries can lead to health and safety initiatives being regarded as unrealistic and impracticable (Fingret and Smith, 1996, p. 16). For example, the UK Manual Handling Regulations, 1992, which followed the European Community's Framework Directive on Health and Safety at Work, is not always fully enforced in hospitals (BMA, 1994). For care workers in domestic settings the monitoring of health and safety standards is more complex and even less likely to take place than in hospitals. Provision of equipment which might prevent injury is more costly, and less likely to be provided. Similarly, unpaid carers are less likely to have access to aids and equipment which are vital to their health and wellbeing.

Changes in employment practices also mean that the boundary between paid and unpaid work is increasingly blurred. Leat and Ungerson note the development of 'flexible labour' in community care in Britain, where workers are expected to work outside 'normal' working hours, to be able to respond as the need arises, and to work unsupervised in people's own homes. They argue: 'the fact that so many of these care workers are women working on their own leads to confusion as to whether this care work is more like informal care, which has traditionally been unpaid, than formal care – which has traditionally been paid' (Leat and Ungerson, 1994, p. 262).

The policy context of caring is varied and often ambiguous. On the one hand, unpaid carers may be regarded as consumers of health and community care services. On the other hand, carers' work is perceived to have value in that it saves public money. In some countries there has been a shift in perception (Millar and Warman, 1996). In Sweden and Norway, for example, some carers have limited rights as formally employed, paid workers (Johansson and Sundstrom, 1994; Lingsom 1994) but this is unusual. In Britain, unpaid carers are entitled to an assessment of their needs under the 1995 Carers Recognition and Services Act but as, Evandrou points out, 'recognition of carers' needs does not necessarily translate into meeting carers' needs' (Evandrou, 1996, p. 228). Tester (1996) notes that, in many European countries, there is reluctance to provide help 'in case this leads family carers to reduce their effort' (Tester, 1996, p. 87). This leaves unpaid carers in an invidious position, valued for what they do but expected to carry on without support and with no rights as consumers of services. As discussed earlier, it is this kind of experience that can lead to poor mental health in carers.

Cultural and religious influences shape expectations about family obligations. In many countries cultural norms of family obligations are deeply entrenched and there is little formal provision to support carers (Salvage, 1995). In Scandinavian countries, despite comprehensive state provision for disabled people, a culture of family obligation persists (Waerness, 1990). Support for carers is, therefore, influenced both by the availability of resources and by prevailing cultural norms about family responsibilities.

Developments in equal opportunities for disabled and older people are an important aspect of the context of caring. The disability lobby has pressed for the right of disabled people to control the way they are supported in living independently. Wilson (1996) argues that Canada, Australia and the USA are far ahead of Europe in achieving a legal framework to promote equal opportunities for disabled people. Again, legal rights do not necessarily entail the provision of adequate resources. In Quebec, for example, the system of 'direct allocations' through which disabled people receive funds to pay their own carers has provided opportunities for greater independence and control by disabled people. However, the level of carers' pay is very low, leading to concerns about exploitation (Stryckman and Nahmiash, 1994). This is not to suggest that the needs and rights of carers and disabled people are inevitably conflicting but that both sets of needs can only be realised by the provision of adequate resources (Morris, 1997; Ungerson, 1997).

Occupational health for carers: implications for policy and practice

Paid and unpaid carers share a great deal in common in terms of the tasks they perform, the conditions in which they work, the nature of their roles and the context in which they carry out their responsibilities. The development of occupational health knowledge and practice, therefore, needs to take into account the whole spectrum of caring. What, then, are the key policy issues arising from this discussion?

First, policy makers need to recognise the direct health effects arising from both the physical environment of caring and the tasks involved. These risk factors also apply to unpaid care. For example, lifting and assistance with mobility as well as contact with toxic substances have been singled out as particularly likely to cause problems for carers working in people's homes. However, financial pressures mean that employers and community care service agencies are unlikely to address these risks.

Second, policy makers need to recognise that the home is a place of work. While it could be argued that an assessment of risks to health in the home is an intrusion on the privacy of the person who is cared for, where the home is a place of work there needs to be a compromise between rights to privacy and rights to health and safety. Finding ways of negotiating such a compromise poses a challenge to health and social services professionals but there are obvious benefits for the person cared for, since the home would become a safer place to live in.

Third, policies need to recognise the emotional as well as the physical impact of caring on health. The experiences of different groups of paid and unpaid carers needs to be taken into account. Co-resident carers, for example, appear to be more likely than other groups to experience 'burn-out', whether the carer is paid or not.

The ability to exercise control over hours worked and having adequate breaks from work have been found to be essential to good health. This poses a challenge to the idea of 'respite' as a service for unpaid carers. Respite emphasises the notion of self-sacrificing vocation in caring whereas the notion of essential breaks prioritises the health of the carer as a worker and also draws attention to the links between working conditions and the quality of the work performed.

These direct effects of caring form only part of the picture of carers' occupational health needs. It is also important to understand the wider context in which caring takes place. As we have seen, the relationship between the carer and the person cared for can influence carers' feelings about their role. Nolan *et al* (1996) refer to the benefits of mutuality in caring relationships. They argue that when carers feel no satisfaction in their role there are serious risks to the safety and wellbeing of both the carer and the person cared for.

It is important therefore that policies recognise the need for carers to exercise choice. The relationship between the carer and outside agencies can significantly affect the wellbeing of carers. Twigg notes that when family members adopt the identity of carers 'it often marks a shift towards a more assertive attitude to the negotiation of public recognition and support' (Twigg, 1994, p. 292). The responses of service providers may either limit or facilitate carers in asserting their needs and negotiating their roles.

This chapter has argued for a recognition of the similarities between paid and unpaid caring as well as an acknowledgement of occupational health problems particular to unpaid care. However, this alone will not transform the experiences of unpaid carers, since occupational health legislation in paid employment is frequently not enforced. It may not be possible to remove all risks and stresses from caring work. However, the health and safety of carers needs to be addressed in policies for developing care in the community. A more complete assessment of the risks faced by carers would reveal more about the true costs of community care. In addition, raising the profile of occupational health hazards could have a beneficial impact on the relationship between service agencies and carers. Health and safety standards provide criteria against which negotiations about caring responsibilities and tasks can be conducted. Caring, like many other occupations contains risks, but policies which are informed by a more thorough knowledge of these would support carers in their attempts to exercise greater control over their work and to assert their rights to health and safety at work.

References

Arber, S. and Ginn, J. (1995) 'Gender differences in informal caring', *Health and Social Care in the Community*, **3**: 19–31.

Ashton, I. and Wright, I. (1995) 'Research in occupational health' in S. Pantry (ed.), *Occupational Health*. London: Chapman & Hall.

Atkin, K. and Rollings, J. (1996) 'Looking after their own? Family care-giving among Asian and Afro-Caribbean communities' in W.I.U. Ahmad and K. Atkin (eds), *'Race' and Community Care*. Buckingham: Open University Press.

Baldock, J. (1997) 'Social care in old age: more than a funding problem', *Social Policy and Administration*, **31**(1): 73–89.

Baldock, J. and Ely, P. (1996) 'Social care for elderly people in Europe: the central problem of home care' in B. Munday and P. Ely (eds), *Social Care in Europe*. Hemel Hempstead: Harvester Wheatsheaf.

Barnett, R. and Marshall, N. (1991) 'The relationship between women's work and family roles and their subjective wellbeing and psychological distress' in M. Frankenhaeuser, U. Lundberg and M. Chesney (eds), *Women, Work and Health: Stress and Opportunities*. New York: Plenum.

British Medical Association (1992) *Stress and the Medical Profession*. London: BMA.

British Medical Association (1994) *Environmental and Occupational Risks of Health Care*. London: BMA.

Caring Costs Alliance (1996) *The True Cost of Caring: A Survey of Carers' Lost Income*. London: Caring Costs Alliance.

Chappell, N.L. and Penning, M. (1996) 'Behavioural problems and distress among caregivers of people with dementia', *Ageing and Society*, **16**: 57–73.

Daykin, N. (1990) 'Health and work in the 1990s: towards a new perspective' in P. Abbott and G. Payne (eds), *New Directions in the Sociology of Health*. London: Falmer.

Dennerstein, L. (1995) 'Mental health, work and gender', *International Journal of Health Services*, **25**(3): 503–9.

Doyal, L. (1995) *What Makes Women Sick: Gender and the Political Economy of Health*. Basingstoke: Macmillan.

Drew, E. (1995) 'Employment prospects of carers of dependent adults', *Health and Social Care in the Community*, **3**(5): 325–31.

Evandrou, M. (1996) 'Unpaid work, carers and health' in D. Blane, E. Brunner and R. Wilkinson (eds) *Health and Social Organisation: Towards a Health Policy for the 21st Century*. London: Routledge.

Evers, A. (1994) 'Payments for care: a small but significant part of a wider debate' in A. Evers, M. Pils and C. Ungerson (eds).

Evers, A., Pijl, M. and Ungerson, C. (eds) (1994) *Payments for Care: A Comparative Overview*. Aldershot: Avebury.

Fingret, A. and Smith, A. (1995) *Occupational Health: A Practical Guide for Managers*. London: Routledge.

Hancock, R. and Jarvis, C. (1994) *The Long Term Effects of Being a Carer*. London: Age Concern Institute of Gerontology.

Hirst, J. (1996) 'A fresh start', *Community Care*, **1127**: 18–19.

Hochschild, A.R. (1983) *The Managed Heart: Commercialization of Human Feeling*. Berkeley, CA: University of California Press.

Hogman, G. and Pearson, G. (1995) *The Silent Partners: The Needs and Experiences of People who Provide Informal Care to People with a Severe Mental Illness*. Kingston-upon-Thames: National Schizophrenia Fellowship.

Joel, M.E. and Martin, C. (1994) 'France' in A. Evers, M. Pijl and C. Ungerson (eds).

Johansson, J.L. and Sundstrom, G. (1994) 'Sweden' in A. Evers, M. Pijl and C. Ungerson (eds).

Leat, D. (1990) *For Love and Money: The Role of Payment in Encouraging the Provision of Care*. York: Joseph Rowntree Foundation.

Leat, D. and Ungerson, C. (1994) 'Great Britain' in A. Evers, M. Pijl and C. Ungerson (eds).

Lingsom, S. (1994) 'Norway' in A. Evers, M. Pijl and C. Ungerson (eds).

Lunn, J.A. and Waldron, H.A. (1991) *Concerning the Carers: Occupational Health for Health Care Workers*. London: Heinemann.

McLaughlin E.(1994) 'Ireland' in A. Evers, M. Pijl and C. Ungerson (eds).

Messing, K. (1994) 'Danger: women at work', *The Women's Review of Books*, **XI**(10–11): 11–13.

Messing, K., Dumais, L. and Romito, P. (1993) 'Prostitutes and chimney sweeps both have problems: towards full integration of both sexes in the study of occupational health', *Social Science and Medicine*, **36**(1): 47–55.

Millar, J. and Warman, A. (1996) *Family Obligations in Europe*. London: Family Policy Studies Centre.

Morris, J. (1997) 'Care or empowerment? A disability rights perspective', *Social Policy and Administration*, **31**(1): 54–60.

National Audit Office (1996) *Health and Safety in NHS Acute Hospital Trusts in England*. London: Stationery Office.

Nolan, M., Grant, G. and Keady, J. (1996) *Understanding Family Care*. Buckingham: Open University Press.

O'Donovan, O. (1997) 'Love labour Irish style' in A. Cleary and M. Treacy (eds) *The Sociology of Health and Illness in Ireland*. Dublin: University College Dublin Press.

OPCS (1992) 'General Household Survey: carers in 1990', *OPCS Monitor Social Survey, 92:2*. London: HMSO.

Parker, G. (1992) 'Counting care: numbers and types of informal carers' in J. Twigg (ed.) *Carers: Research and Practice*, London, HMSO.

Parker, G. and Lawton, D.(1994) *Different Types of Care, Different Types of Carer: Evidence from the General Household Survey*. Social Policy Research Unit. London: HMSO.

Rantalaiho, L.(1997) 'Contextualising gender' in L. Rantalaiho and T. Heiskanen (eds), *Gendered Practices in Working Life*. Basingstoke: Macmillan.

Sainsbury, D. (1994) 'Women's and men's social rights: gendering dimensions of welfare states' in D. Sainsbury (ed.), *Gendering Welfare States*. London: Sage.

Salvage, A.V. (1995) *Who Will Care? Future Prospects for Family Care of Older People in the European Union*. Dublin: European Foundation for the Improvement of Living and Working Conditions.

Smith, P. (1992) *The Emotional Labour of Nursing*. London: Macmillan.

Stryckman, J. and Nahmiash, D. (1994) 'Canada' in A. Evers, M. Pijl and C. Ungerson (eds).

Tancred, P. (1995) 'Women's work: a challenge to the sociology of work', *Gender, Work and Organisation*, **2**(1): 11–20.

Taylor, R., Ford, G. and Dunbar, M. (1995) 'The effects of caring on health: a community-based longitudinal study', *Social Science and Medicine*, **40**(10): 1407–15.

Tester, S. (1996) *Community Care for Older People: A Comparative Perspective*. London: Macmillan.

Thomas, C. (1995) 'Domestic labour and health: bringing it all back home', *Sociology of Health and Illness*, **17**(3): 328–52.

Twigg, J. (1994) 'Carers, families, relatives: socio-legal conceptions of caregiving relationships', *Journal of Social Welfare and Family Law*, **16**(3): 279–98.

Twigg, J. and Atkin, K. (1994) *Carers Perceived: Policy and Practice in Informal Care*. Buckingham: Open University Press.

Ungerson, C. (1994) 'Morals and politics in "payments for care": an introductory note' in A. Evers, M. Pijl and C. Ungerson (eds).

Ungerson, C. (1997) 'Give them the money: is cash a route to empowerment?', *Social Policy and Administration*, **31**(1): 45–53.

Waerness, K. (1990) 'The rationality of caring' in C. Ungerson (ed.), *Gender and Caring: Work and Welfare in Britain and Scandinavia*. New York: Harvester Wheatsheaf.

Warner, N. (1995) *Better Tomorrows: Report of a National Study of Carers and the Community Care Changes*. London: Carers National Association.

Warren, L. (1990) '"We're home helps because we care": the experience of home helps caring for elderly people' in P. Abbott and G. Payne (eds), *New Directions in the Sociology of Health*. London: Falmer.

Wilson, V. (1996) 'People with disabilities' in B. Munday and P. Ely (eds), *Social Care in Europe*. London: Prentice Hall, Harvester Wheatsheaf.

4 HEALTH AND WORK IN THE SEX INDUSTRY

Graham Scambler and Annette Scambler

This chapter continues with the theme of socially constructed notions of work and their restrictive impact on the scope of occupational health research and practice. The authors examine a particular form of invisible work: voluntary adult sex work in modern western societies. While this is not taken to represent all forms of sex work, it can be seen as an example of a form of unrecognised and unregulated work with attendant unaddressed health risks. The authors explore the extent to which the application of currently accepted definitions of work to this activity would highlight the problems faced by sex workers as well as identifying the day to day strategies that they, like other workers, employ to protect themselves from hazards. Redefining prostitution as 'work' may strengthen the case for the decriminalisation of prostitution and the extension of citizenship rights to sex workers, thus facilitating the development of more effective health promotion strategies. However, it would not necessarily fully reflect the complex nature of sex work and may even limit understanding of some of its dimensions. The authors highlight some of these dimensions which include power, patriarchy, exploitation and choice as well as changing forms of sexuality. These lie outside conventional discourses of work and risk but they are important to an understanding of the nature of work in the sex industry.

The issues surrounding the substitution of the phrase 'sex work' for 'prostitution' are important and contentious, not least for the consideration of matters of occupational health, the central concern of this book. The increasingly widespread tendency to refer to sex work, for example, has been associated with a more systematic interest in attendant 'occupational health problems'. For some critics, the term sex

71

work lends dignity and legitimacy to a thoroughly flawed and unacceptable social institution, while for others it acknowledges that its practitioners sell services (not themselves) in a distinct, if lonely and sometimes hazardous and threatening, marketplace. This chapter explores such issues, drawing especially on our own and others' research in the health domain. In the opening section we offer a brief social profile of sex workers in 'high' modernity, stressing the naive and erroneous nature of popular stereotypes. We then describe the legal status of sex workers in England and Wales, showing its salience for their health experience and behaviours. This is followed by a discussion of the concept of sex work, and by a consideration of conditions of work and of health and safety. The closing section focuses on the importance of 'operational', 'political' and 'structural' change for the health and wellbeing of sex workers.

Sex workers

The term 'sex industry' is used to cover many kinds of labour. In this chapter we shall focus on what might be called 'voluntary adult sex work' in modern western societies. However, it is important to recognise from the outset that involuntary (forced, coerced) or under-age prostitution, sometimes linked to sexual tourism, is also an extremely common phenomenon. Altink (1995) is among those who have documented contemporary sexual trafficking and slavery, abusive health-exacting and even life-threatening forms of prostitution that have all been widely condemned, but arguably are increasing in a high modernity characterised by new and readily accessible global rather than national markets and an associated refiguring of time and space. Issues of legal jurisdiction and policing in relation to such phenomena have become extremely complex (see Edwards, 1997).

The most common stereotypical image of the prostitute or sex worker in modern western society is probably that of a woman wearing a miniskirt and high heels offering her services to kerb-crawling motorists from the backstreets of a big city. She may also be deemed coarse, uneducated, a heavy alcohol or drug user and suffering from problems of mental health or maladjustment originating in early parental or other abuse (Barbara, 1993). While there are sex workers who fit this description, they are exceptional. Moreover street workers in general constitute only the conspicuous tip of an iceberg, with perhaps as many as nine out of ten sex workers conducting their business, more or less discreetly, 'indoors' (Boyle, 1994).

Pheterson (1993) has systematically debunked many of the myths associated with women sex workers. Elsewhere we have built on her insights by proposing acceptance of five propositions about this heterogeneous population (Scambler, 1997; Scambler and Scambler, 1998). The first of these insists, against popular stereotypes, that most women sex workers are neither vulgar nor immoral; nor do most live or work in milieux characterised by habitual drug use, violence, anomie and hopelessness. In fact, most women in the industry are inconspicuous or 'hidden' off-street workers, many of them able to avoid public labelling (and even self-labelling) as misfits and outsiders. They are for the most part 'ordinary' rather than 'extraordinary'.

Second, it is neither accurate nor warranted to characterise women sex workers as passive 'victims' of socio- or psychopathological background circumstances. There is no reason to believe them to be less active and independent than any other group of female workers. Not only do they frequently require considerable drive and initiative to work safely and successfully, but they may exercise a greater degree of control during their encounters with clients than many other female workers. They should therefore be seen as active, autonomous agents unless and until there is evidence to the contrary.

Third, there is no justification for assuming that women sex workers lack moral sensibility or commitment. It is evident from numerous ethnographic accounts that women commonly develop their own codes of practice to govern a range of work-related and health-protecting behaviours from condom use to sexual services. Nor is it appropriate to assume that they are any more predisposed to infringe social norms or laws – other than those prohibiting or constraining their work practices – than other people.

Fourth and relatedly, the pragmatic skills, expertise and resourcefulness of women sex workers should not be underestimated. Most women learn quickly of the demands and hazards of sex work, and no less rapidly have any preconceptions they might have had about the hypocrisy and fallibility of 'respectable' men reinforced. Their reflexivity and agency therefore needs to be stressed.

Finally, there is an innovative aspect to women sex workers' norm-breaking which is often neglected. Giddens (1992) has suggested that a new potential to challenge patriarchal structures and ways of thinking has arisen recently through a combination of factors, including 'plastic sexuality'. Plastic sexuality refers to sexuality liberated from its intrinsic relation to reproduction. Its emergence was a precondition, he maintains, of the sexual revolution, with its 'gains' in female sexual autonomy and a flourishing of gay culture. These gains constitute a considerable challenge to what Brittan (1989) calls 'hierarchic heterosexuality'.

A more audacious claim might be that women sex workers manage to integrate plastic sexuality with the reflexive project of self. It is autonomy and reciprocity that are crucial here. Certainly some women, although by no means all, choose the rewards of sex work, like higher pay than most women and many men aspire to in more orthodox employment, foreign travel and unusual freedom over working hours; and some enjoy (aspects of) their work (French, 1988). Moreover, although the industry remains symptomatic of patriarchy, this does not prevent most women from controlling most of their encounters with most of their clients: there is resistance to patriarchy even here.

These theses amount to a contention that it be presumed that women sex workers are individualistic, active and wilful, moral, reflexive and resourceful, as well as possible innovators in relation to the norms of hierarchic heterosexuality. What cannot be denied, however, is that some women, perhaps a small minority, conform precisely to the stereotype of the sex worker. Nor should it be forgotten that selling sexual services can be dangerous, leave emotional scars and, in exceptional circumstances, lead to death.

Sex work and the law

The nature and extent of the laws governing sex work are of crucial importance for occupational health because they constrain the perceptions and behaviours of both sex and health workers. While there are societies in which sex work is prohibited by law – witness most states within the USA for example – most seek to discourage and constrain rather than to ban it. The basic legal parameters in England and Wales are paradigmatic in this respect and therefore worth considering in some detail. The most significant Acts are the Sexual Offences Act 1956, the Street Offences Act 1959 and the Sexual Offences Act 1985.

In modern western societies legislation around the sex industry, and even more so police and court enforcement of legislation, has been concerned above all else with curtailing visible street work (Darrow, 1984). In England and Wales, for example, the Street Offences Act 1959, which outlawed loitering and soliciting, precipitated an immediate but temporary decline in street activity and numbers of women prosecuted (although this may in large part have been a function of changes in police procedures and powers (Edwards, 1987). In 1982 the Criminal Justice Act abolished imprisonment for loitering and solic-iting, a reform that may have been related to prison overcrowding rather than to humanitarianism. This appears to have encouraged more women to work on the streets.

The considerable increase in prosecutions for loitering and soliciting through the 1980s – 12 per cent in London, for example, between 1981 and 1989 (Personal communication, Home Office, 1992) – has generally been attributed both to the 'tough policing' congruent with the ethics of the New Right, and, perhaps more significantly, to addi-tional women turning to sex work due to an erosion of other employ-ment opportunities and welfare support. The English Collective of Prostitutes (ECP) (1988) estimated that 70 per cent of women sex workers are supporting children. Since imprisonment for loitering and soliciting was abolished in 1982, heavier fines have been imposed. This has had two effects: women have felt compelled to return to the streets to pay off their fines, and the rate of imprisonment for fine defaulting has risen steadily (Edwards, 1987).

The policing of street work is costly of scarce resources that some police officers judge could be better invested elsewhere. But the police are not always free to exercise discretion and are frequently obliged to attempt to enforce sections of the Street Offences Act by local authori-ties or residents' associations. However they are aware that heavy or saturation policing leading to cautions and arrests for loitering and soliciting, or tactics like no parking zones or one-way road systems to inhibit kerb crawlers, merely subdue or displace street activity for a while. The disruption of street activity leads inevitably to the disrup-tion of strategies – usually painstakingly evolved and deployed – by health workers to distribute health education literature and condoms and to persuade sex workers to attend mobile or local out-patient clinics for health checks, advice or support.

The Sexual Offences Act 1985 proscribed kerb crawling. The 1989 statistics for London revealingly show only one client prosecution for kerb crawling or persistent soliciting of a woman sex worker under this Act for every 69 prosecutions for loitering or soliciting under the Street Offences Act 1959. Yet Morgan Thomas (1992) has estimated that clients probably outnumber women sex workers by at least 50:1.

It has been suggested that the Sexual Offences Act 1985 owed more to the lobbying of professionals anxious to protect their wives and daughters and maintain the respectability of their neighbourhoods than it did to any impulse to 'equalize' the legal response to women sex workers and their clients. Certainly the Act was opposed by the ECP and others. Its effect was similar to that of the Street Offences Act

1959, making trade more difficult for women accustomed to working the streets, obliging many of them either to make more instant, and therefore potentially more hazardous, judgements about the trustworthiness of clients with cars or to find alternative ways of contacting them (Edwards, 1987).

The Sexual Offences Act 1956 was directed against third-party profiteers. The 1989 statistics, however, show only 30 magistrate and 40 crown court prosecutions under the Act for living off the earnings of women sex workers or exercising control in London (Personal communication, Home Office, 1992). It is not known what proportion of women sex workers in London are directly managed or controlled, although vice-squad officers estimate that in most red-light districts approaches are made to almost all street workers after they begin working (Boyle, 1994).

In Birmingham, in 1982, it was estimated that 75 per cent of all women sex workers have pimps (McLeod, 1982). Estimates like these highlight the degree of immunity from prosecution managers or controllers enjoy. The Sexual Offences Act 1956 may in fact threaten unemployed kin or cohabitees who can be shown to be profiting from the earnings of sex work, while being largely ineffective against the more vicious pimps it was primarily designed to deter or punish. This problem has been acknowledged by the Criminal Law Revision Committee but not yet been effectively addressed.

Sex 'work'

It is appropriate here to refer to what we have elsewhere defined as the *paradox of attention* (Scambler, 1997). This states that much of the notoriety and excitement evoked by prostitution or sex work is a function less of what sex workers actually do than of the fascination it has for others. It is apparent, for example, that many of the objections to sex work, feminist and non-feminist, apply equally well to alternative forms of work to which far less attention and ire is directed. In fact, women sex workers lead lives more prosaic and mundane than is suggested in the excesses of attention and stereotype. For the most part they are ordinary women systematically and ideologically misrepresented – in line with the projects of those who do so – as extraordinary.

They may be employed by others or self-employed; they may work full time, part time or casually (as when they temporarily tread the city streets in the weeks prior to Christmas to earn the money for their children's presents); they may work from the streets, in hotels, saunas or massage parlours, in brothels, from escort agencies, or from their own or others' flats; they may experience rigid dependency on others or substantial independence and autonomy; they may be safe or protected or exposed and at risk; but, however heterogeneous their backgrounds and circumstances and conditions of work, they attract pay for services often not in themselves illegal and, indeed, are potentially liable for taxation on their earnings. Whichever property of sex work is highlighted is neither exclusive to that form of work nor the object of such attention and interest in relation to other forms of labour.

As far as recruitment is concerned, there are numerous factors which predispose to sex work, but perhaps the most obvious is relative poverty. McLeod (1982) characterises women's entry to the sex industry as an act of resistance in the face of the experience or threat of relative poverty. Perkins and Bennett (1985) report that 97 per cent of the women they sampled in an Australian survey gave money as their principal motivation for becoming sex workers, and 95 per cent of these spoke in terms of 'economic survival'. Some have claimed that recruitment is almost exclusively 'from the working class and the lumpenproletariat' (Hoigard and Finstad, 1992, p. 15), but this is to oversimplify.

Certainly personal biography is salient: women sex workers are more likely than non-sex workers to have had poor relationships with their fathers and, to a lesser extent, to have been abused by them; to have grown emotionally distanced from their families of origin and thus from family disapproval and influence; and to have developed strong and independent personalities. As McLeod (1982, p. 30) insists, however, if personal biography does predispose to sex work, it does so only in association with local conditions, 'such as the existence of a number of women working in prostitution and more structural forces such as employment opportunities'. Peer contact can be an important feature of recruitment.

A neglected group of women, proportionately more of them from middle-class backgrounds and working off-street, appear to have 'consciously chosen' sex work. Deploying the concept of choice here – and referring to 'voluntary adult sex work' – remains contentious. Certainly choices have to be interpreted in the context of the psychosocial circumstances in which they are made. Nevertheless, there are women who claim to have consciously chosen sex work (and not always solely in preference to unemployment or underemployment) for its extrinsic rewards in terms of money, autonomy or travel (Perkins and Bennett, 1985), and some (even) for its intrinsic satisfaction and enjoyment (French, 1988).

Women's patterns of work are partly determined by type and location of work: thus the routines of street workers, hotel or bar workers,
workers in saunas or massage parlours, workers with escort agencies
and workers in flats and brothels all differ and with a degree of consis-
tency. The reference to 'routines' here is apposite, since for many
women in the sex industry work tends towards a dull and sometimes
inebriated monotony characterised by a great deal of waiting around
(Connie: 'whoring is boring, but lucrative', quoted in Taylor, 1991,
p. 17; and see Jaget, 1980).

Sex workers are far from unique in finding much of their work
monotonous. Nor are they exceptional in developing instrumental attitudes to both work and their clients. Typically, their priority is to draw
encounters to a conclusion in the shortest manageable time ('A good
customer is a fast customer'); many cut themselves off mentally for the
duration of contact ('I try to think of something else, plan what I am
going to do with the money'); and many, too, forbid the intimacy of
kissing and see the condom as a barrier, real and symbolic ('He will
never be able to reach me, I think to myself. It is like the condom guar-
antees that he will never touch me') (Jarvinen, 1993, p. 144). Once
again, however, we must be wary of broad generalisations: the instrumental approach defined here may be pervasive (as well as commended
as 'professional' within the industry), but caring for clients, especially
regulars, is not unknown, nor (even) are orgasms with clients
(Jarvinen, 1993).

The range and nature of the services requested and provided within
the sex industry are enormous, only some of them having to do with
genital sex. Frequently women evolve their own 'code of practice'
which extends beyond an insistence on hygiene and condom use and
proscribes sexual (and other) acts outside a pre-defined set of categories. Many women will not participate in or sanction acts which
they see as deeply degrading: 'As a prostitute you've got to be comfortable with what you take on, otherwise it becomes too stressful. If you
keep on pushing yourself into situations which you dread or find
repulsive then you do suffer psychological damage' (quoted in Silver,
1993, p. 87).

Fees for services are as variable as work patterns. Boyle's (1994)
observation that women who work independently, inconspicuous and
underrepresented in research studies, tend to enjoy the highest
incomes is probably correct. Boyle (1994, p. 145) records the rates
charged by Samantha, typical of those paid to workers on the streets or
women 'working the windows': '£10 for hand relief, £15–20 for
straight sex, £20 for oral, £25 for oral and sex or strip and sex, £30 for

strip, oral and sex, and those wanting to spend 30 minutes of their time with her will have to fork out £40.' These rates may be compared with those of another interviewee, Diana, a 30-year old occupant of a mews cottage close to London's Regents Park. About 95 per cent of Diana's work is 'specialised': a dominatrix, her work revolves around fantasy and S&M. For clients unsure what they want she provides a 'taste of everything' over a 90-minute session for £500. Despite considerable overheads, she clears up to £1500 profit a week. It is perhaps part of the stereotype of the sex worker that any attempt to accumulate money to finance a subsequent respectable and comfortable lifestyle is doomed to fail: women supposedly neither save nor emerge from the sex industry unscathed. This view is reinforced by research on the experiences of ageing, drug-using or otherwise 'trapped' sex workers. But there is, of course, a dearth of research on women – be they full-time, part-time or occasional casual workers – who have saved and left the industry without scars to return incognito into the community.

Health and safety

Conventionally, prostitutes or sex workers have been regarded as purveyors of disease (see Walkowitz, 1980). They have attracted the attention of health researchers and policy makers to the extent that their (immoral) behaviours have been defined as constituting a 'risk' to other (normal, moral) citizens. To define the selling of sexual services as a form of work or labour is to adopt an entirely different and more fruitful perspective. As Chapkis (1997, p. 57) observes, it is then the context and conditions of work that become paramount. She writes:

> Those who are enslaved (i.e. coerced by 'traffickers') must be made free either to leave the trade or to join those who are 'merely' exploited in demanding better wages, safer working conditions, and greater control over the labour process. Such a perspective allows prostitution to be examined critically as a form of service work, with attention focused on factors enhancing or limiting a worker's power relative to clients, employers and colleagues. When erotic labour is viewed as work, it is transformed from a simple act of affirmation of man's command over woman, and instead is revealed to be an arena of struggle, where the meaning and terms of the sexual exchange are vulnerable to cultural and political contestation.

The epidemiological 'surveillance' conducted in relation to women sex workers since the mid-1980s has led to a less alarming picture than many moral entrepreneurs anticipated. A multicentre cross-sectional survey of women sex workers across nine European countries reported an overall prevalence rate for HIV infection of 1.5 per cent in non-intravenous drug users and 31.8 per cent in intravenous drug users (European Working Group on HIV Infection in Female Prostitutes, 1993). Seventy-nine London women were included, three of whom were intravenous drug users; none tested positive. In a larger London series, prevalence rates for HIV of 1.7 per cent for 1986–88 and 0.9 per cent for 1989–91 were found (Barton *et al.*, 1987; Day *et al.*, 1988; Ward *et al.*, 1993). Infection in these women was related to injecting drug use or to sex with non-paying partners known to have HIV.

Rates of HIV infection outside London vary (Scambler and Scambler, 1997), but it seems clear that women who inject drugs and share equipment experience an enhanced risk, and that those who do not inject may also be at risk through sexual intercourse, either with clients or with non-paying partners. Ward *et al.* (1993) found that the proportion reporting always using condoms for vaginal sex with clients rose from just under half in 1985 to 98 per cent in 1990. Condom use tends to be lower with regular than with casual clients, and lowest with non-paying partners. Given that some partners may be injecting drug users and/or be having unprotected sex with other women, it may be, paradoxically in light of moral panics fostered by the media, that while clients generally remain protected through consistent condom use, women sex workers are at risk of HIV infection from their partners. Since condoms are as important as symbolic barriers between women and their clients as their absence is crucial to establishing intimacy with non-paying partners, there appears to be no straightforward solution to this problem.

Ward *et al.* (1993) found rather higher rates of other sexually transmitted infections: 44 per cent of their sample in 1980–91, for example, reported a past history of gonorrhoea. In Sheffield, Woolley *et al.* (1988) found that 28 per cent of women had at least one episode of gonorrhoea during 1986–87, and 24 per cent had chlamydia.

Health problems other than sexually transmitted diseases include drug use and injury or abuse. The use of tobacco and illicit drugs like cannabis by women sex workers can be high. In Edinburgh, for example, it was discovered that 87 per cent of women sex workers smoked; of those who had consumed alcohol in the week before the study, the mean consumption was 48.1 units (one unit being equivalent to half a pint of normal strength beer, lager or stout or to a single bar-room measure of spirits or to a glass of wine); 93 per cent of women had smoked cannabis, and a third had at some stage used heroin (Morgan Thomas, 1990; Plant, 1990). Plant (1997) has attributed these high rates to a variety of factors: for example, in some environments women engage in sex work to pay for drugs, and conditions of work in the sex industry can of course fuel the use of substances. Drug use in Edinburgh, however, may be unusually high.

Injury and abuse are far from uncommon, especially for street workers. It has even been suggested that sex work is 'very often about violence' (Barnard, 1993). McKeganey and Barnard (1996) found violence against women working the streets of Glasgow commonplace; they add, however, that although violence was reported by almost all women, only a minority of client encounters involved violence. Attacks are rarely reported to the policy (Scutt, 1994), with women largely dependent on their own strategies: taking control of encounters, using intuition born of experience, adopting working rules, liaising with other workers, and carrying weapons.

Mention should be made finally of women sex workers' general health needs, that is, those they share with non-sex workers. Although it is reasonable to assume that their general health status may be poorer than that of non-sex workers, especially in the case of street workers, because of the unpredictable, stigmatizing and often stressful nature of their work, there is as yet no direct evidence of this.

The challenge of health-enhancing change

Almost all the efforts made so far to improve the health status of women sex workers have been at what we have elsewhere called the *operational level*; and, arguably, these have amounted to little more than exercises in damage limitation (see Scambler and Scambler, 1995). Operational change refers to health promotion or service initiatives directed by health workers or other experts, at the public or at key groups or key settings which neither challenge nor threaten core social institutions.

In contrast, changes at the *political level* involve initiatives which bear on health but are beyond the influence of health workers. Ultimately the intervention of government is required. Change at this level brings core social institutions into focus and may, typically indirectly, challenge or threaten them. Change at the *structural level* is deeper yet: this refers to fundamental revisions within core social institutions which bear on health but which are beyond the capacities of both health workers and parliamentary governments to deliver. Change at the structural level typically requires a mobilization of mass public support which, in turn, typically requires sustained and organised extra-parliamentary political action.

Drawing on these distinctions we have elsewhere offered a fairly radical agenda for change under the general rubric of health promotion (Scambler and Scambler, 1995, 1998). At the operational level we have advocated a shift in the orientation of health education and prevention work in acknowledgement that the sex industry embraces not only sex workers but also clients, who may outnumber sex workers by at least 50:1, and third parties such as brothel managers, pimps and law enforcement agencies (Morgan Thomas, 1992). Many sex workers are already active in health education and prevention, especially concerning safer sex practices with clients; they should no more be cast as passive recipients than judged to be the sole targets of such programmes (Kinnell, 1989).

Politically, health education initiatives need to be directed, we have maintained, at government agencies. We have highlighted two principles objectives here. The first is the de-criminalisation (not legalisation) of sex work through the abolition of those laws pertaining exclusively to prostitution, a reform which might be defined as a form of health protection (see Downie et al., 1990). Accompanying this reform should be moves to extend normal citizenship rights to women in the sex industry, from welfare benefits to tax liability.

The second political objective involves a programme, in so far as it lies within the compass of government agencies to sustain one, to reverse the growth of relative poverty among women generally and single mothers in particular (Lister, 1992). Such a programme, an example of health protection on numerous counts, would mitigate against involuntary recruitment to the sex industry (independently of its legal status).

As far as structural change is concerned, we advocated a greater awareness and knowledge of the significance of change at the structural level for the distribution of health. Structural change, too, may be a precondition for effective political and operational change. For example, British women's continuing economic and (hierarchic heterosexual) dependencies are an intrinsic part of a 'system of patriarchal institutions, norms and relationships', as are the often isolated, marginal and health-exacting lives of women sex workers (Scambler et al., 1990). Structural change can also constitute a form of health protection.

In many ways this agenda amounts to a push for the recognition of prostitution as sex 'work'. It is proffered with conviction and without apology but with full acknowledgement that such a recognition cannot be justified on health grounds alone (Scambler and Scambler, 1997). Accepting the incommensurability of certain feminist readings of prostitution, Chapkis (1997, pp. 213–14) deliberately and instructively adopts a 'hybrid perspective' in order to 'build bridges' across competing analyses and stances. It is a perspective which 'draws on the strengths of conflicting accounts', incorporating the insistence that injustice must be challenged rather than accommodated; the insight that subversion is a creative ally to opposition; the recognition that simply because something appears to have 'always' existed it is neither inevitable nor unchangeable; and a reminder to the advocates of 'prostitutes' rights' that transformation does not reduce to a politics of prohibition.

A feminist politics rooted in such a hybrid perspective, she suggests, might permit a pragmatic consensus around three key goals. The first of these is a basic redistribution of wealth and power between, as well as among, men and women. Gross economic disparity stratified by class, gender, ethnicity and nation-state, Chapkis insists, leads to conditions of economic coercion that undermine meaningful 'choice'. 'No woman should be forced to engage in prostitution – or any other form of productive or reproductive labour – against her will.' The second goal centres around an organised and empowered workforce and the need to generate policies geared to workers' interests, rather than those of employers or clients. 'Prostitutes, as all others who labour for a living, should be guaranteed full workers' rights and benefits.' Third, there should be a decriminalisation of adult consensual sexual activity. The state, Chapkis maintains, should not criminalise adult sexual behaviour, whether in the context of 'loving relationships, recreational encounters or commercial transactions'. Rather, 'our collective resources should be devoted to teaching respect for sexual diversity and creating conditions under which consent can be made more meaningful.' Whether Chapkis offers what amounts to an effective strategy for accomplishing the 'broad-based feminist alliance' necessary to achieve such an ambitious triad of goals might be debated. She certainly does not minimise or understate the obstacles.

It is in our view important to distinguish between voluntary adult sex work and involuntary (forced, coerced) or under-age prostitution, for reasons which have been apparent throughout the present discussion (see also Chapkis, 1997, pp. 41–57). Axiomatically, however, if the former, as sex 'work', were to survive into a world no longer stratified by class, gender, ethnicity and nation-state, it would and could bear scant resemblance to the contemporary sex industry.

Perhaps the most important single conclusion arising from our own enquiries in the health domain is that sex workers are, and are likely to remain, only minimally responsive to orthodox 'individualised' health service and promotion strategies – that is, to strategies within the compass of operational change – while they continue precariously to occupy positions on the political and structural margins of society.

References

Altink, S. (1995) *Stolen Lives: Trading Womem into Sex and Slavery*. London: Scarlet Press.

Barbara (1993) 'It's a pleasure doing business with you', *Social Text*, **37**: 11–22.

Barnard, M. (1993) 'Violence and vulnerability: conditions of work for street working prostitutes', *Sociology of Health and Illness*, **15**: 693–705.

Barton, S., Taylor-Robinson, D. and Harris, J. (1987) 'Female prostitutes and sexually transmitted diseases', *British Journal of Hospital Medicine*, **7**: 34–45.

Boyle, S. (1994) *Working Girls and their Men: Male Sexual Desires and the Fantasies Revealed by the Women Paid to Satisfy Them*. London: Smith Gryphon.

Brittan, A. (1989) *Masculinity and Power*. Oxford: Blackwell.

Chapkis, W. (1997) *Live Sex Acts Women Performing Erotic Labour*. London: Cassell.

Darrow, W. (1984) 'Prostitution and sexually transmitted diseases' in K. Holmes, P. Mardh, P. Sparling and P. Weisner (eds), *Sexually Transmitted Diseases*. New York: McGraw-Hill.

Day, S., Ward, H. and Harris, J. (1988) 'Prostitute women and public health', *British Medical Journal*, **297**: 1585.

Downie, R., Fyfe, C. and Tannahill, A. (1990) *Health Promotion: Models and Values*. Oxford: Oxford Medical Publications.

ECP (1988) *Women Prostitutes and Aids: Resisting the Virus of Repression*. London: English Collective of Prostitutes.

Edwards, I. (1987) 'Prostitutes: victims of the law, social policy and organized crime' in P. Carlen and A. Worrell (eds), *Gender, Crime and Justice*. Milton Keynes: Open University Press.

Edwards, S. (1997) 'The legal regulation of prostitution: a human rights issue' in G. Scambler and A. Scambler (eds), *Rethinking Prostitution: Purchasing Sex in the 1990s*. London: Routledge.

European Working Group on HIV Infection in Female Prostitues (EWGHFP) (1993) 'HIV in European female sex workers: epidemiological link with use of petroleum-based lubricants', *AIDS*, **7**: 401–8.

French, D. (1988) *Working: My Life as a Prostitute*. London: Gollancz.

Giddens, A. (1992) *The Transformation of Intimacy: Sexuality, Love and Eroticism in Modern Society*. Cambridge: Polity.

Hoigard, C. and Finstad, L. (1992) *Backstreets: Prostitution, Money and Love*. Cambridge: Polity.

Jaget, C. (ed.) (1980) *Prostitutes: Our Life*. Bristol: Falling Wall.

Jarvinen, M. (1993) *Of Vice and Women: Shades of Prostitution*. Scandinavian Studies in Criminology, Vol. 13. Oslo: Scandinavian University Press.

Kinnell, H. (1989) *Prostitutes, their Clients and Risks of HIV Infection in Birmingham*. Occasional Paper. Birmingham: Department of Public Health Medicine.

Lister, R. (1992) *Women's Economic Dependency and Social Security*. Manchester: Equal Opportunities Commission.

McKeganey, N. and Barnard, M. (1996) *Sex Work on the Streets: Prostitutes and their Clients*. Buckingham: Open University Press.

McLeod, E. (1982) *Working Women: Prostitution Now*. London: Croom Helm.

Morgan Thomas, R. (1990) 'AIDS risks, alcohol, drugs and the sex industry' in M. Plant (ed.) *AIDS , Drugs and Prostitution*. London: Routledge.

Morgan Thomas, R. (1992) 'HIV and the sex industry' in J. Bury, V. Morrison and S. McLachlan (eds), *Working with Women with AIDS: Medical, Social and Counselling Issues*. London: Routledge.

Perkins, R. and Bennett, G. (1985) *Being a Prostitute: Prostitute Women and Prostitute Men*. Sydney: Allen & Unwin.

Pheterson, G. (1993) 'The whore stigma: female dishonour and male unworthiness' *Social Text*, **37**: 39–54.

Plant, M. (1990) 'Sex work, alcohol, drugs and sex' in M. Plant (ed.), *AIDS, Drugs and Prostitution*. London: Routledge.

Plant, M. (1997) 'Alcohol, drugs and social milieu' in G. Scambler and A. Scambler (eds), *Rethinking Prostitution: Purchasing Sex in the 1990s*. London: Routledge.

Scambler, G. (1997) 'Conspicuous and inconspicuous sex work: the neglect of the ordinary and mundane' in G. Scambler and A. Scambler (eds), *Rethinking Prostitution: Purchasing Sex in the 1990s*. London: Routledge.

Scambler, G., Peswani, R., Renton, A. and Scambler, A. (1990) 'Women prostitutes in the AIDS era', *Sociology of Health and Illness*, **12**: 260–73.

Scambler, G. and Scambler, A. (1995) 'Social change and health promotion among women sex workers in London', *Health Promotion International*, **10**: 17–24.

Scambler, G. and Scambler, A. (1997) 'Afterword: rethinking prostitution' in G. Scambler and A. Scambler (eds), *Rethinking Prostitution: Purchasing Sex in the 1990s*. London: Routledge.

Scambler, G. and Scambler, A. (1998) 'Women sex workers, health promotion and HIV' in S. Kendall (ed.), *Health and Empowerment Research and Practice*. London: Arnold.

Scutt, J. (1994) 'Judicial vision – rape, prostitution and the chaste woman', *Women's Studies International Forum*, **17**: 345–56.

Silver, R. (1993) *The Girl in Scarlet Heels*. London: Century.

Taylor, A. (1991) *Prostitution: What's Love Got to do With It?* London: Macdonald.

Walkowitz, J. (1980) *Prostitution and Victorian Society*. Cambridge: Cambridge University Press.

Ward, H., Day, S., Mezzone, J., Dunlop, L., Donegan, C., Farrar, S., Whitaker, L., Harris, J. and Miller, D. (1993) 'Prostitution and risk of HIV: female prostitutes in London', *British Medical Journal*, **307**: 356–8.

Woolley, P., Bowman, C. and Kinghorn, G. (1988) 'Prostitution in Sheffield: differences between prostitutes', *Genitourinary Medicine*, **64**: 391–3.

5 DEATH AND INJURY AT WORK: A SOCIOLOGICAL APPROACH[1]

Theo Nichols

The following chapter examines different perspectives on the causes of occupational ill health, focusing in particular on industrial accidents and injury rates. The author explores the nature of risk discourses which have shaped occupational safety management and regulation. Apparently neutral, official voices have in fact tended to give disproportionate weighting to various forms of methodological individualism in the analysis of injury rates. Hence the psychology or behaviour of individual workers has often been the focus of attention, while the social and economic determinants of accidents have been played down or ignored. There is clearly a need to redress this imbalance. In highlighting the importance of social processes of causation linked to factors such as the business cycle, industry characteristics, social relationships and political strategies, Theo Nichols demonstrates the importance of the contribution that the social sciences can make to occupational health research.

According to World Health Organisation and International Labour Office estimates, there are about 120 million workplace accidents a year worldwide and about 200,000 deaths. The Health and Safety Executive (HSE) recently attempted to estimate the cost in Britain. The HSE assumed approximately 500 fatal injuries; in addition, almost three-quarters of a million injuries which led to absence from work of over three days; and at least one and a half million injuries which led to absence for part of a day or longer. Absence due to injury was put at a minimum of eighteen million days lost, in the region of ten times the days lost by strikes (*Employment Gazette*, December 1994, p. S42). For employers alone, the cost of personal injury at work was estimated at approaching a thousand million pounds in 1990 prices (Davies and Teasdale, 1994, pp. vi, 16). This does not take account of any suffering or financial loss by employees.

Understanding and preventing industrial injury

Among social scientists the early contributions to the study of industrial injury came from psychology in the shape of research into accident proneness. This goes back to the investigations into injuries incurred by British women munitions workers in the First World War carried out for the Industrial Fatigue Research Board (Greenwood and Woods, 1919). They had found that many women munitions workers had no accidents, some had one, but others had as many as five in a period of thirteen months. The Board declared in a review of its work up to 1921 that 'Greenwood and Woods, by the statistical treatment of accident records kept by certain munitions factories, have adduced evidence to show that accident incidence... depends largely on some quality of susceptibility inherent in the personality of the victims' (Industrial Fatigue Research Board, 1921, p. 23). It was not too difficult to determine what to do about this unfortunate problem, especially since some believed that there was also 'some indication that those prone to industrial accidents are industrially inefficient'.

In keeping with the spirit of scientific management the accident proneness concept was picked up by a whole wave of industrial psychologists in the USA who searched for the causes of accidents in the psychology of individual workers (Berman, 1978, p. 23). Today the explanation of industrial accidents in terms of 'accident proneness' is widely rejected on methodological grounds. Psychologists increasingly make their contribution through research into the perception of risk, often converging with those working within the sociology of organisations. However, notions about the personality of the victim live on.

Assumptions about individual behaviour and choices as determinants of industrial injury have also influenced economic perspectives on safety at work. The inspiration for many in this area goes back to Adam Smith and his theory of compensatory wage differentials: 'the wages of labour vary with the ease or hardship, the cleanliness or dirtiness, the honourableness or dishonourableness of the employment' (1970, Book One, Chapter 10). The truth is of course the opposite. To quote J. S. Mill in his *Principles of Political Economy* (1965): 'The really exhausting and really repulsive labours, instead of being better paid than others, are almost invariably paid the worst of all, because performed by those who have no choice.' In practice, the modern economist, just like Adam Smith himself, adds a qualification – that the compensatory element applies, other things being equal. But despite this, any assumptions about 'free choices' existing for workers must be treated with care.

By contrast, the sociological study of industrial injury, especially from the standpoint of political economy, shifts the focus away from the individual/victim. It emphasises that people do not make their choices in circumstances that are of their own choosing, and it holds that these circumstances merit examination in their own right, particularly the social and political relations in which they are enmeshed.

Official observers often fail to recognise the social determinants of industrial injury. The influential Robens Report on Safety and Health at Work in the UK, for example, which came out in 1972, attributed accidents to 'apathy'. This followed a long established if ill grounded conventional wisdom. The Industrial Fatigue Research Board had similarly noted, in 1922, that 'machinery is responsible for only a minority of accidents which occur in factories and workshops... a great number of such accidents are due simply and solely to carelessness, inattention, and want of thought' (Industrial Fatigue Research Board, 1922, p. v). This showed, so the Research Board concluded, that the 'importance of the personal factor has been officially recognised'. The notion that 88 per cent of all accidents are primarily produced by the 'human factor' had also been substantially publicised by Heinrich, whose application of scientific management to safety engineering goes back to his *Industrial Accident Prevention: A Scientific Approach* first published in the United States in 1931.

The problem is, as another sociologist has said of Heinrich, 'from the moment the human factor is considered to be the cause of accidents, everything the worker does and omits to do can be blamed. In this way a definition can be arrived at in which nearly all accidents are attributed to the worker' (Dwyer, 1991, p. 148). In practice it is increasingly recognised that there is little in work organisations that does not depend on the human factor or ultimately lead back to management. However, the emphasis on the human factor has a long history and is generally used to mean just 'the worker'. In my view, sociologists have a contribution to make here, but they must go beyond both the 'human factor' and simple notions of 'choice'. Economic and political trends as well as labour market conditions and developments in technology all need to be examined in terms of their influence on workers' health.

Injury rates and the business cycle

Although business cycles are not God given in either their magnitude or
frequency and do not have God-given effects either, they do tend to have
a relation with the manufacturing injury rate. Intuitively, it would
appear likely that there might be an anti-cyclical relation. As the cycle
goes up employment increases and managements find labour more of a
scarce resource. Workers, on the other hand, feel more confident about
protecting their health and safety. These two sets of factors might be
expected to send injuries down. Conversely, when the cycle goes down,
unemployment goes up, workers are less able to protect themselves,
management pushes harder and injuries might be expected to rise.

In fact, the relation is, if anything, the opposite. This can be seen
approximately in Figure 5.1, where the engagement rate is used as a
proxy for the business cycle. On reflection, there are several processes
that may be at work in the upturn which lead to more injuries. More
inexperienced workers are taken on who are particularly at risk; yet
despite this increased recruitment, management fails to maintain the

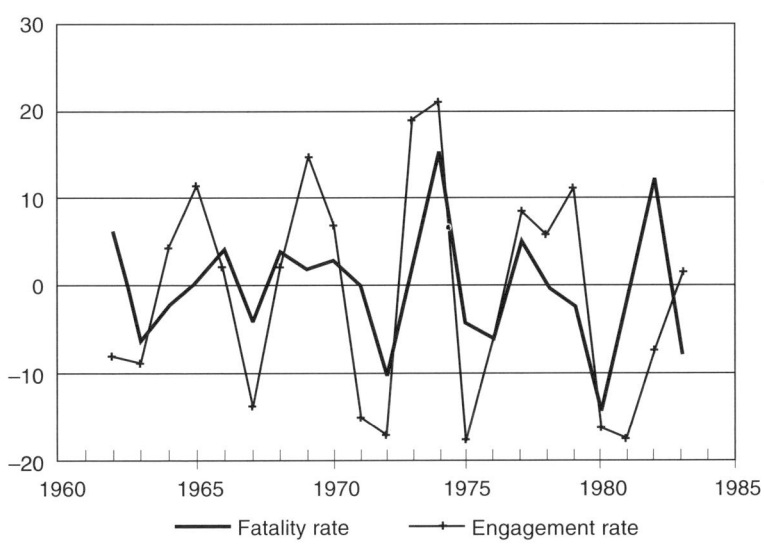

Figure 5.1   Employee fatality and engagement rates: deviations
from the trend, 1960–85

Source: Nichols, 1989b

previous labour/output ratio, so that the intensity of work increases. Depending on the basis for the calculation of the injury rate, increased injury rates may also be caused because more overtime is worked or because more workers are taken on in higher risk occupations than lower risk ones. In the case of a cyclical downturn, all these processes are likely to operate the other way round with a decline in economic activity being accompanied by a decline in injury rate. Two things to notice are first that these processes make better sense of injury rate fluctuation than does the idea that 'apathy' goes up and down; and second that many of these changes take place despite the attitudes of individual managers and individual workers in the sense that they are not consciously related to safety.

What is being suggested here is that there is scope for a wider socio-logical approach to industrial injury, one that speaks to the structures and dynamics of economy and society, which takes the form of an economic sociology or political economy, and which lies outside the conventional wisdom and notions of the 'human factor' and 'apathy'. This has been developing since the 1970s when research on the shop floor began to locate the causes of accidents in the social relations of production (Nichols and Armstrong, 1976). This form of analysis can give a very different impression to that conjured up when 'attitudes' are invoked in a politico-economic void. In particular, it suggests that rather than arising from the interruption of the production process, injuries may often result from attempts to 'keep the job going'.

American research has confirmed this view through an examination of accident reporting in a Texas limestone quarry (Perrow, 1984). The worker concerned was doing his usual eleven-hour shift, which consisted of shovelling away the crushed limestone that had fallen underneath a four-foot wide conveyor belt. The material was hard to remove from under the belt, and there was no provision for stopping the belt. Whereas the Mine Safety and Health Administration (MSHA) investigators concluded that 'the victim had crawled under the conveyor while it was running for unknown reasons', the researcher himself makes some quite different observations: that 'an obvious known reason would be that [crawling underneath the conveyor] was the only way to prevent the materials from building up to where it would damage the conveyor belt – which was, after all, his job'; that 'one might truly say that this was a "forced error"...if the operator did not keep the... area clean, one strongly suspects, he would be forced to look for another job'; and that the incident 'gives us some idea of what most people in the accident business mean when they classify such accidents as "operator error"' (Perrow, 1984, pp. 246–9). This example underlines the inappropriateness of using the term 'accident' which indicates a random event, or one without cause. This man was doing his job, which was part of a regular, structured activity. For this reason, there is a growing preference among health and safety activists not to use the term 'accident' but to address the causes of injuries themselves. It is, as Marx clearly saw, the workers' capacity to labour that is purchased by capital. All is are not dotted and all ts are not crossed in advance of work being actually performed. Testimony to the extent to which, day by day, managements are dependent on workers' initiative is the rapidity with which production can grind to a halt if they work to rule. Of course workers, even with the best of intentions, can get it wrong. This was well illustrated at the US nuclear power station at Three Mile Island, where operators, faced with both inadequate instrumentation and multiple alarms, intervened at an early stage, but in fact made decisions which made the situation worse.

Management sometimes relies more than it cares to admit on the fact that workers will intervene. Relevant here is another example from the nuclear power industry (provided by Hale, 1985). When the Central Electricity Generating Board (CEGB) applied for planning permission to build the first British pressurised water reactor (Sizewell B), part of its safety case was that the reactor would shut itself down automatically after a loss of coolant, without even requiring the operator to intervene until 30 minutes after the incident. Critics pointed out at the public enquiry that this only eliminated operator errors of omission. It did not allow for errors of commission as at Three Mile Island. It was then suggested that, if plant shutdown really could be achieved in all cases without human intervention, it would be logical to lock the operators out of the system during this half hour. This suggestion was resisted. There were still, it was said, eventualities where it would be advantageous if the operator could intervene to improve upon the performance of the automated system. It was also accepted that unforeseen situations could occur beyond the design base of the automatic system, where the human being would be the final line of defence.

The politics of industrial injury

During the 1980s the idea that British workers were holding down productivity, a long standing refrain of both Labour and Tory governments, was aggressively revived. The Thatcher government made some extraordinary claims – that it had turned round productivity, achieved growth rates reminiscent of Japan, and cured 'the British disease'.

However, these achievements – such as they were – rested much less on the deepening of investment in plant and in people and more on the weakening of labour by economic, political and ideological means. In manufacturing industry, these policies spelt the intensification of labour which in turn spelt increased danger for workers, as did the anti-regulatory climate and the fetishisation of markets.

It is therefore important to examine the effects of the Thatcher regime on industrial injury. Did the expected deterioration show up in the injury rate as manufacturing itself, in the official version, got leaner and fitter? Research suggests that it did (Nichols, 1986b). Between 1981 and 1984 manufacturing industry's major injury rate (which measures serious injuries such as fractures and amputations) increased by nearly 25 per cent. The increase was widespread. It occurred in 15 of the 17 SIC Orders which made up manufacturing industry. As can be seen from Figure 5.2, the fall in the fatality rate in manufacturing was also checked at about this time (Nichols, 1986b).

As the economy began to recover from the massive blow dealt to it during the early years of the first Thatcher government, a number of

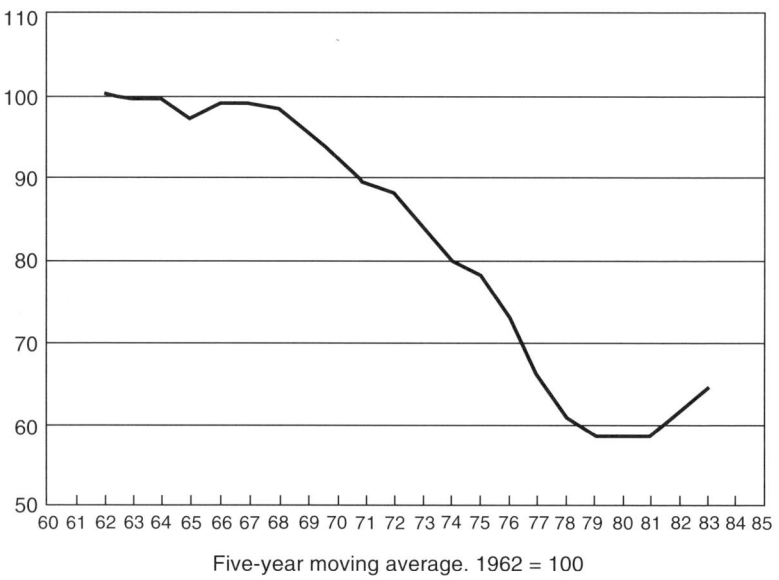

Five-year moving average. 1962 = 100

Figure 5.2   Trend of employee fatality rate in British manufacturing, 1960–85

Source: Nichols, 1989b

corner-cutting and labour-intensifying processes exacted their toll. There was a variety of adaptations to the new economic and political climate such as reductions in washing-up time and in tea breaks and increases in flexibility. At the same time work was delivered more regularly and constantly to workers' workstations. This was seen by managements as making the workplace 'more efficient', and was sometimes accompanied by a shift from just-in-case to just-in-time systems (see Canaan, this volume). All these processes led to the porosity of the working day being reduced. They were paralleled by decreased working-class confidence to resist and increased uncertainty and fear, and by reductions in maintenance, in housekeeping, in training, and in manning. There was a particular reluctance by managers, who had recently witnessed a sharp economic collapse, to take on new labour as the cycle went up (Nichols, 1991) and workers' health suffered as a result.

The sociology of disasters

Since the early 1980s the world has witnessed a number of disasters or near disasters – in Britain, Piper Alpha in the North Sea and a rash of other well publicised tragedies; elsewhere, Three Mile Island, Chernobyl, above all Bhopal where no one knows the death toll. It is sometimes estimated at 15,000, and life went cheap, at circa $2000 per head, for which Union Carbide sought all possible means to avoid responsibility. All this has fostered interest in man-made disasters and a specialist literature has developed.

The social causes of disasters have been discussed by Turner (1978; 1992). A British engineer turned sociologist, Turner suggests that: 'To the sociological eye, engineering systems are always sociotechnical systems, made up of a technical system embedded within a social system' (1992, p. 186). His aim was to unify the understanding of the seemingly unrelated and indeed irregular and unique events that constitute disasters. Fundamental here is a model in which most system failures are not caused by a single factor and in which conditions for failure do not develop instantaneously. Rather, there is an 'incubation period' when multiple predisposing factors accumulate, unnoticed, or not fully understood. The predisposing factors are then combined into a single occurrence, a trigger event, usually an unanticipated discharge of energy of some kind, which provokes the onset of system failure. This model makes no prediction about the onset of particular disasters (quite reasonably) but nor is there any central proposition about the development of disasters over time.

The American sociologist Perrow has a different emphasis to Turner, arguing that information systems are becoming less able to cope with developments in high technology. In particular, he argues that there is now a greater threat from accidents that 'involve the unanticipated interaction of multiple failures' (1984, p. 70). His concern is primarily about the catastrophic potential of high risk technologies. He argues these will inevitably, and increasingly, produce accidents because of the difficulty of designing out the occurrence of unexpected interactions among two or more failed components. We have accidents such as at Three Mile Island, Perrow argues, because we have built an industrial society that has some parts that, like industrial plants or military ventures, have highly interactive and tightly coupled units (1984, p. 8). The complexity and coupling of high technology means that another Three Mile Island is only a matter of time.

Despite the increased sociological interest in disasters, the general run of industrial injuries continues to be subject to a series of commonplace hand-me-down questions. Who has been careless? Who was apathetic? Who chose to work in a job because of the good money? Isn't it, after all, a macho job? Who neglected to wear their goggles/gloves/visor? And, quintessentially, with reference to the *Herald of Free Enterprise*, who left the bow doors open?

Working conditions and workers' responses to occupational injury

A recent example of blaming the victim comes from Australia and relates to the so-called epidemic of reported cases of repetitive strain injury (RSI) which occurred between the mid-1970s and 1980s (see Canaan, this volume). This was depicted as being nothing more than an expression of the 'Australian worker problem' or alternatively 'kangaroo paw' or 'golden arm' as some Australian commentators called it, given the implications for compensation. Some RSI sufferers were additionally subject to a barrage of racist ideology expressed in jibes about 'Mediterranean back', 'Lebanese wrist' and 'Greek back'. The concentration of immigrant men and women workers in sectors that required continuous and repetitive tasks gave these attacks a superficial credibility.

In Australia the debate was heightened by the presence of unionised workforces, and relatively highly developed and active women's campaigns and health and safety movements. It was also intensified by a compensation system in which court cases were initiated by employers in order to shed liability for workers already on compensation. Hence these employers were encouraged to cast doubt on the existence of injury. Quinlan and Bohle (1991) have pointed out that RSI is not an Australian phenomenon, and the 'epidemic' had understandable causes. Nor in fact, for the record, is RSI either mainly a white-collar phenomenon, or a new one, with reports of 'telegraphists' cramp' in Britain going back to 1875.

Behind the talk of kangaroo paw lies a generally negative view of industrial injuries, the idea of the 'pseudo accident' or the 'not truly accidental accident'. In British social science these ideas can be traced back to the 1960s, to the work conducted by the Tavistock Institute for Human Relations, which was influenced by the psychoanalytic approach of Melanie Klein (Nichols, 1994), and to the work on industrial injury rates by the sociologist Baldamus (1971). Among other things, Baldamus looked at the effects of accidents by days of the week, and at the effects of piecework wages. But what is important for the argument here is that he also distinguished between reported injuries of different degrees of severity.

He observed that in the 1960s rates for more and less severe injuries behaved differently. Minor injuries rose when the others did not. He concluded that there was a sociological explanation for this which had to do with the changing structure of employment opportunity and changes in expectations. He held that there were underlying processes at work, which, in particular circumstances, expressed themselves in a higher reported injury rate. This is reflected over the 1960s in data on the reported incidence of sprains and strains, on the one hand, and of fractures on the other (Figure 5.3).

There are at least two ways of understanding this. One is exemplified in headlines such as 'Lying Workers Cost Us Millions' (Nichols, 1975). The other is that what we have here is some sort of seismograph of worker confidence. This allows the possibility that some people do pretend to be injured when they are not; but also that many people carry minor injuries and aches and pains pretty well by the day, so that the decision to take time off to recuperate is a sociologically variable one. This accords well with Baldamus's argument that a variety of different factors will influence workers' decisions to take time off.

Differential propensity to take time off for injury may also play a part in generating different patterns of injury between different sections of the working population. A comparison between the self-employed and employees is instructive here. As far as major injuries are concerned the pattern of injury is much the same for each of these groups. Whether we look at the self-employed or at the employed, 75 per cent of their major injuries are fractures. However, minor injuries are a different matter.

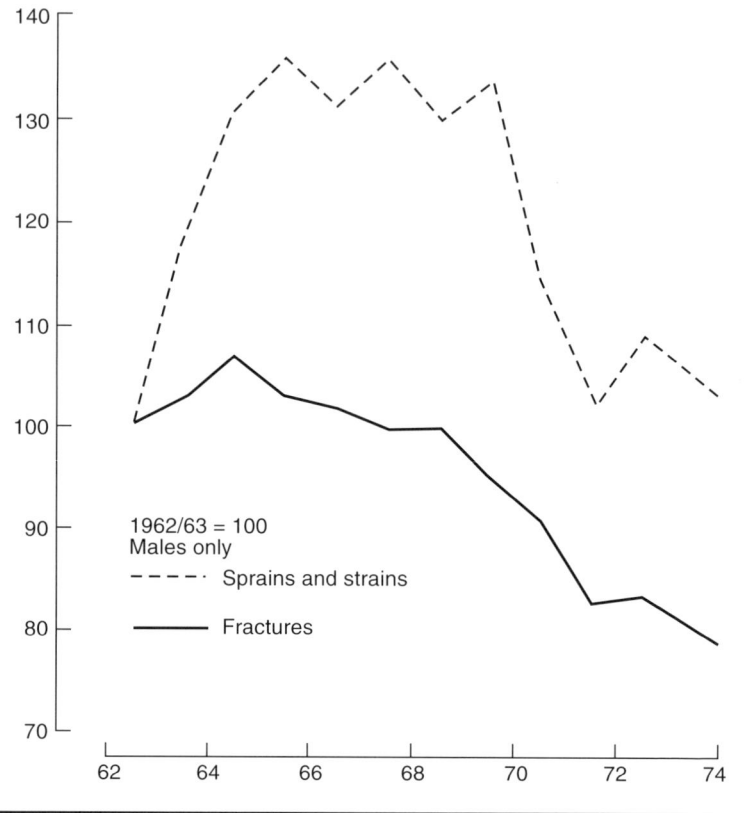

Figure 5.3   Causes of certified incapacity for injury benefit,
1962/63–1974/75

Source: Nichols, 1989b

For the self-employed, strains and sprains make up less than 20 per cent of minor injuries; for the employed the figure rises above 40 per cent. There is no warrant to conclude from this that employees are malingering. On the contrary, 'self-employed' individuals may often have less real choice when it comes to taking time off to recuperate from injury and to safeguard their health. However, there is certainly something here to be explained. The best response is not to say that these injury rates are just socially constructed, but to ask what is going on, how, why and with what consequence? A further implication is that if we want to assess safety over time, it is better not to look to minor rates of injury, which are the most affected by differential propensity to take time off.

Small is beautiful? The effects of business size on industrial injuries

The structural location of employed people – whether they work in small or large employment units for instance – also has significant consequences for injury rates. The case that small is beautiful has been argued in at least three different ways specifically with respect to industrial injury (Hopkins and Palser, 1987). In fact each of these different theories turns on assumptions about the nature of bureaucracy. First, there is the morale theory, which argues that large size means bureaucratisation and bureaucracy spells low morale. Second, there is the worker autonomy theory, which claims that large size means bureaucratisation and bureaucracy spells a lack of worker autonomy, which itself leads to increased injury. Third, there is the argument that injuries are a function of poor communications, which are again assumed to stem from bureaucracy, which is again assumed to be a function of size. The information in Figure 5.4 is in line with this broad general position and would seem to suggest that small *is* beautiful.

However, my own research on British manufacturing in the early 1980s suggested an alternative view based on the idea of 'structures of vulnerability'. This argued that industries typified by the presence of small rather than large establishments would tend to undergo the greatest *deterioration* in safety during the period 1981–84. In other words, both the assumptions and the findings about size and safety were just the opposite of the relation implied in Figure 5.4. Moreover, the HSE later confirmed that there is an association between small size and higher injury rates.

Recently, a secondary analysis of the Workplace Industrial Relations Survey – the national ED/ESRC/PSI survey of what is happening to industrial relations in Britain – has provided a better basis for the examination of associations with size than HSE's own data. Figure 5.5 shows quite clearly that the injury rate is higher in smaller establishments. Indeed, further analysis suggests that the injury rate is *higher* in small establishments whether they are independent establishments (separate small businesses) or whether they are part of larger organisations. Generally, the bigger, the more beautiful, and the smaller the less so – the opposite of the conclusion suggested before.

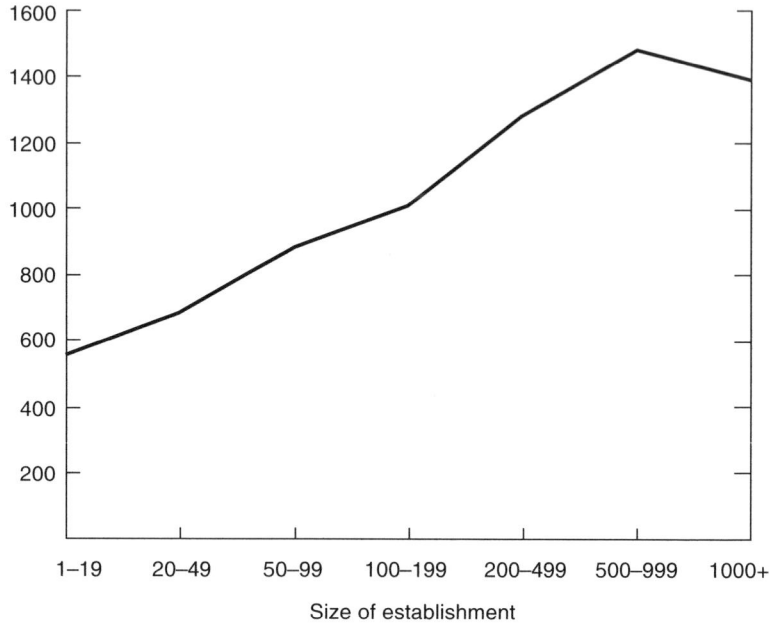

Figure 5.4   Minor injury rate per 100,000 employees and
size of establishment

Source: Nichols *et al.*, 1995

How are these different results to be explained? The answer lies in
the fact that the injury rates in Figures 5.4 and 5.5 measure different
things – minor and major injuries respectively (see Figure 5.6).

The positive association between small size and low injury rate – the
small is beautiful idea – is found in relation to the minor injury rate.
Among other things, this is likely to be explained, at the level of micro
politics by a greater vulnerability of the employee *vis-à-vis* the
employer, which makes it more difficult to take time off. Another causal
factor is likely to be the pronounced absence of trade unions in small
establishments. But whether small employers are more likely to be
authoritarian or not, the lower level of minor injuries in small establishments is also likely to be an outcome of the fact that loss of labour is
more critical in small establishments than in larger ones. The smaller
the unit, the more any reduction in number hurts the employers.

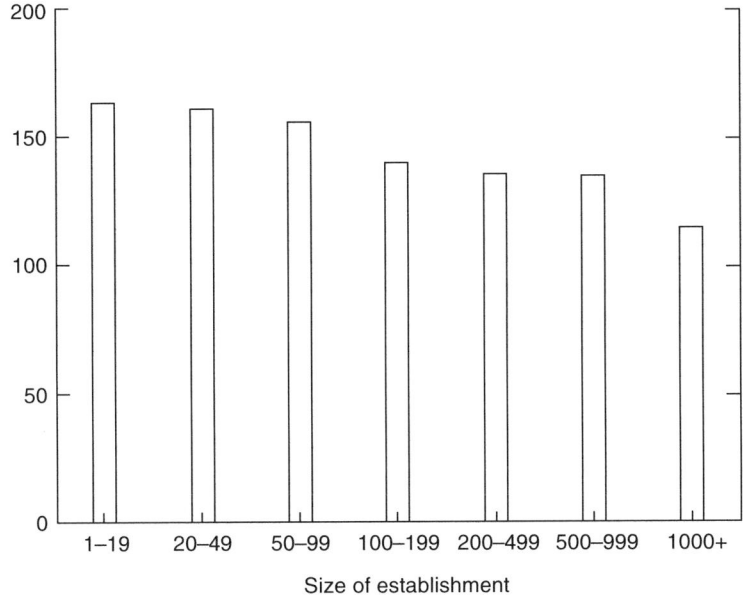

Figure 5.5   Major injury rate per 100,000 employees and
size of establishment

Source: Nichols *et al.*, 1995

The negative association – the small is dangerous idea – holds in
relation to the major injury rate and resources are crucial here. Bigger
establishments generally have greater resources to put into training.
They also tend to have more for investment, are more able to ride out
hard times, are less inclined to corner cutting. They are more likely to
be unionised and to have safety committees.

There is much more that could be said about this (Nichols *et al.*,
1995; Nichols, 1997). One interesting aspect of the relationship
between small size and injury is that the smaller the plant the longer
the time period it will take for any given rate of injury to affect a plant
employee. In other words, the relatively greater danger of small establishments may lie outwith the experience of those who work for
themand indeed of those who manage them. But the point is this:
minor injury rates are more affected by propensity to take time off:

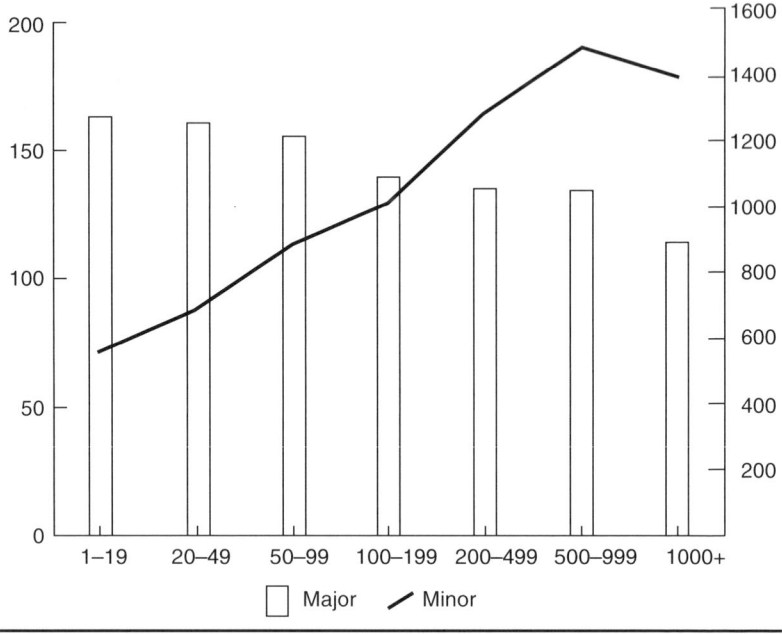

Figure 5.6   Injury rate per 100,000 employees and
size of establishment
Source: Nichols *et al.*, 1995

major rates of injury are better indicators of safety. And, where safety is concerned, small is *not* beautiful.

It is important to establish that small plants are more dangerous given the development of a new trend in thinking about the industrial future. Some social scientists have recently put forward prescriptions for a new manufacturing pattern based on small workshop strategies, the so-called flexible specialisation strategy. One of the damaging consequences for labour of this rather romantic view would probably be a higher injury rate. Less fanciful has been the tendency for governments to promote cutting so-called health and safety 'red tape' which purportedly 'burdens' small business.

Technology, progress and improvements in workers' health

Space does not allow for an examination of the complexities of the relationship between trade unionism and safety, or of the possibilities of safety committees and participation, or of different payment systems, or of different forms of employment relation. Nor can we explore the role and past effectiveness of the law in safety regulation. All of these matters are of importance and require further sociological investigation (a task attempted in Nichols, 1997). They touch on how we organise economic, social and political relations, and on how this relates to some of us getting hurt at work.

However, there is space for consideration of one final issue, that of the implications of technological developments for improving workers' health. The advertisement in Figure 5.7 about Sir Humphry Davy and his safety lamp captures what used to be the progressive line on science and technology. It is the antithesis of this progressive vision that I will be addressing here, with specific reference to the history of major injury. This antithesis has been captured as well as anyone by Douglas Coupland in a word introduced in his fictional commentary on the generation that was born between 1961 and 1971, the so-called *Generation X* of his book's title. The word is 'cryptotechnophobia': the secret belief that technology is more of a menace than a boon.

It is not uncommon, for instance, for writers on industrial accidents and safety to claim that the introduction of the Davy lamp – which earlier generations had been told by their history teachers saved miners' lives – actually led to more miners being killed (Albury and Schwartz, 1993). As the modern version of the Davy parable goes, Davy was called in by the mineowners in the north east of England, not to save miners' lives, but in order that they could profit by working seams that otherwise could not be worked because of the risk of methane explosion. There are three things to say about this.

First, it is probably true that more miners died in the fifteen years after the introduction of the Davy lamp than in the fifteen years before. Second, it is true that the lamp was developed out of considerations of profit. Had the priority been to save miners lives, money would have been put into the ventilation system, since miners were not dying from explosion but from suffocation. However, there is something that modern accounts do not always make clear. Although 20 per cent more miners were killed in the fifteen years after the introduction of the Davy lamp than in the fifteen years before, nearly 40 per cent more miners were employed in the later period (compare for example the accounts by Albury and Schwartz, 1982, 1983 and Hair, 1968). Given that the *rate* of fatal injury therefore went down, it is not as straightforward as is sometimes implied to dismiss the safety lamp's contribution to safety.

HUMPHRY DAVY. HIS LAMP WAS ONE OF THE ORIGINAL LIFE SAVING DEVICES

In 1815 a committee was formed in England to prevent explosions in mines. These disasters were caused by methane, which mixed with air and was ignited by miners' candles. Since methane is a colorless, odorless gas its victims had no warning of impending danger.

The committee turned to one of the most famous chemists of the day. Humphry Davy had already successfully challenged Lavoisier's theory of acids, had discovered chlorine and the alkali metals and had done some brilliant work in electro-chemistry.

In studying methane, Davy discovered it had a surprisingly high ignition temperature.

Within three months, he perfected a new lamp which enclosed a flame within cylinder of fine wire mesh. The principle was incredibly simple. In passing through the wire mesh, heat from the flame was cooled to a temperature below methane's ignition point.

The Davy Lamp saved thousands of lives and is one of the earliest examples of how pure science could help industry.

Several years ago a major chemical corporation established its own separate department responsible for Safety, Health and Affairs Related to the Environment. Throughout its operations, from processing plants to every phase of delivery, the people who run SHARE are working with local management to improve the corporation's safety performance and assure the integrity of the air and water at its plants and the surrounding communities.

SHARE's success has dramatized industry's ability to preserve the quality of our lives and its work will continue. After all, Humphry Davy lit a lamp on behalf of humanity and no one wants to see it go out.

Figure 5.7   Advertisement

Source: Chemical and Engineering News, 3 May 1976

From this, I want to suggest a more general point: that the effects of investment-driven productivity on safety are not to be dismissed in advance, either. It is only necessary for example to think of the introduction of microelectronics into production to see that one effect may be to remove workers from exposure to danger in the shape of moving machinery. More generally, it is probable that the incorporation of best practice into technology also tends to improve safety over time.

Figure 5.8 plots information on fatalities and productivity in British coal mines from two readily accessible time series. It can be seen that over this period the British coal industry both improved productivity and reduced the fatality rate. This pattern can be contrasted with that suggested by data on Turkish coal mining (Nichols and Kahveci, 1995). Figure 5.9 shows the course taken by productivity and injury at the Zonguldak coalfield in north west Turkey over almost half a century. Broadly speaking the two move together, not one up and one down. Had there been the same relationship between productivity and injury rate in the British mines as there was in Turkey, between 1947 and 1977 the rate for fatalities would not have fallen by 50 per cent as it did. Rather, it would have risen by about 250 to 300 per cent, with truly devastating consequences for British miners.

In Turkey, productivity and injury moved together. This happened because the mines were starved of investment, with few changes in the labour process over a whole half century, so that higher productivity was a function of, as one miner put it, *insan gücü* (literally 'human-power'); and, because, up to the 1990s the labour movement continued to be weak. There is a lesson here. On the one hand, there is no iron law which makes further technological development lead to reductions in injury over time and occupational health may not improve even if injury rates do. On the other hand, the progressive effects of investment-based technological change on injury do require more acknowledgement than they sometimes receive.

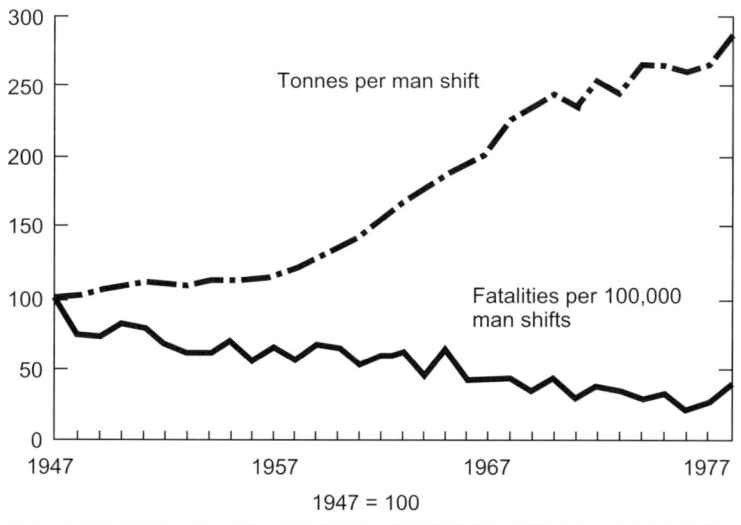

Figure 5.8   Coal production and injuries in British mining, 1947 to 1978/79

Source: Ashworth, 1986, Table A2, pp. 677–81

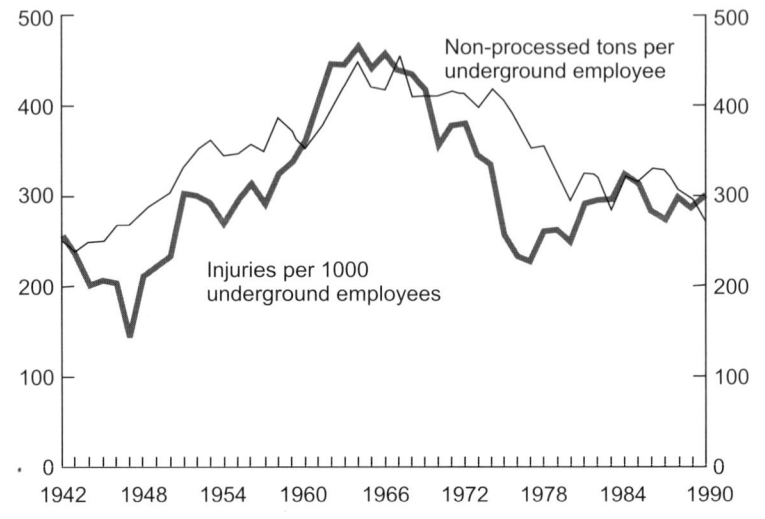

Figure 5.9   Productivity and injury rate, Zonguldak Coalmines,
Turkey, 1942–90

Source: Nichols and Kahveci, 1995

Conclusion

It is fitting to have concluded with reference to a less developed country.
Industrial injuries afflict workers worldwide. Increasingly we all live in
one capitalist world where the heavy and dirty end of production,
including an increasing amount of manufacturing, is located outside
the boundaries of the advanced capitalist states. Indeed partly because
of this and other changes in the internal composition of industry, official injury statistics can make recent overall safety performance in
countries such as Britain appear better than it actually is. And even in
the advanced capitalist states, future improvement in safety performance in the workplace is not assured. In the British case, for example,
it is indicative of current political priorities that at the end of 1994
there were still fewer factory inspectors in post than there had been in
1979. A further deepening of 'Victorian' economic and political structures – more small firms, further reductions in the role of trade unions,
continued mass unemployment and a growth in the self-employed – is
unlikely to make for improved safety in many workplaces.

Note

1. This chapter is based on a public lecture given at the University of Bristol in February 1995. Many of the issues raised are explored more extensively in Theo Nichols (1997) *The Sociology of Industrial Injury*. London: Mansell.

References

Albury, D. and Schwartz, J. (1982) *Partial Progress: The Politics of Science and Technology*. London: Pluto.

Albury, D. and Schwartz, J. (1983) 'Why the safety lamp increased accidents', *New Scientist*, 10 February.

Ashworth, W. (1986) *The History of the British Coal Industry, Volume 5, 1946–1982: The Nationalized Industry*. Oxford: Oxford University Press.

Baldamus, W. (1971) 'The consumption imperative: structural change in advanced capitalist societies'. Discussion Paper E18. Birmingham: University of Birmingham.

Berman, D.M. (1978) *Death on the Job: Occupational Health and Safety Struggles in the United States*. New York: Monthly Review.

Coupland, D. (1992) *Generation X*. London: Abacus.

Davies, N.V. and Teasdale, P. (1994) *The Costs to the British Economy of Work Accidents and Work-Related Ill Health*. London: HSE Books.

Dwyer, T. (1991) *Life and Death at Work: Industrial Accidents as a Case of Socially Produced Error*. New York: Plenum.

Greenwood, M. and Woods, H.M. (1919) 'The incidence of industrial accidents upon individuals with special reference to multiple accidents', Industrial Fatigue Research Board, Report 4. London: HMSO.

Hair, P.E.H. (1968) 'Mortality from violence in British coal mines', *The Economic History Review*, **21**(3).

Hale, A.R. (1985) *The Human Paradox in Technology and Safety*. Delft: Delft University of Technology.

Heinrich, H.W. (1959) *Industrial Accident Prevention: A Scientific Approach*. New York: McGraw-Hill (first published 1931).

Hopkins, A. and Palser, J. (1987) 'The causes of coal mine accidents', *Industrial Relations Journal*, **18**(2) Spring.

Industrial Fatigue Research Board (1921) Second Annual Report to 30 September 1921 (including analysis of published work). London: HMSO (published 1922).

Industrial Fatigue Research Board (1922) *Report 19: Two Contributions to the Study of Accident Causation*. London: HMSO.

Mill, J.S. (1965) *Principles of Political Economy*. Toronto: University of Toronto Press (first published 1848).

Nichols, T. (1975) 'The sociology of accidents and the social production of injury' in G. Esland, G. Salaman and M.-A. Speakman (eds), *People and Work*. Edinburgh and Milton Keynes: Holmes McDougall in association with Open University Press.

Nichols, T. (1986a) 'Industrial injuries in British manufacturing in the 1980s', *Sociological Review*, May.

Nichols, T. (1986b) *The British Worker Question: A New Look at British Workers and Productivity*. London: Routledge & Kegan Paul.

Nichols, T. (1989a) 'On the analysis of size effects and "accidents"', *Industrial Relations Journal*, **20**(1) Spring.

Nichols, T. (1989b) 'The business cycle and industrial injuries in British manufacturing over a quarter of a century', *Sociological Review*, August.

Nichols, T. (1990) 'Industrial safety in Britain and the 1974 Health and Safety at Work Act: the case of manufacturing', *International Journal of the Sociology of Law*, **18**.

Nichols, T. (1991) 'Labour intensification, work injuries and the measurement of percentage utilisation of labour (PUL)', *British Journal of Industrial Relations*, **29**(4).

Nichols, T. (1994) 'Industrial accidents as a means of withdrawal from the workplace according to the Tavistock Institute of Human Relations: a reexamination of a classic study', *British Journal of Sociology*, **45**(3) (September).

Nichols, T. (1997) *The Sociology of Industrial Injury*. London: Mansell.

Nichols, T. and Armstrong, P. (1973) *Safety or Profit: Industrial Accidents and the Conventional Wisdom*. Bristol: Falling Wall.

Nichols, T. and Armstrong, P. (1976) *Workers Divided*. Glasgow: Fontana.

Nichols, T. and Beynon, H. (1977) *Living With Capitalism*. London: Routledge & Kegan Paul.

Nichols, T., Dennis, A. and Guy, W. (1995) 'Size of employment unit and injury rates in British manufacturing: a secondary analysis of WIRS 1990 data', *Industrial Relations Journal*, **26**(1) March.

Nichols, T. and Kahveci, E. (1995) 'The condition of mine labour in Turkey: injuries to miners in Zonguldak 1942–90', *Middle Eastern Studies*, **31**(2), April.

Perrow, C. (1984) *Normal Accidents: Living with High-Risk Technologies*. New York: Basic Books.

Quinlan, M. and Bohle, P. (1991) *Managing Occupational Health and Safety in Australia*. Melbourne: Macmillan.

Smith, A. (1970) *The Wealth of Nations*. Harmondsworth: Penguin.

Turner, B.A. (1978) *Man Made Disasters*. London: Wykeham Publications.

Turner, B.A. (1992) 'The sociology of safety' in D. Blockley (ed.), *Engineering Safety*. Maidenhead: McGraw-Hill.

6 WHY WE STILL HAVE 'OLD' EPIDEMICS AND 'ENDEMICS' IN OCCUPATIONAL HEALTH: POLICY AND PRACTICE FAILURES AND SOME POSSIBLE SOLUTIONS

Andrew Watterson

Following on from the previous analysis of perspectives on industrial injury causation, this chapter takes a closer look at the social processes influencing recognition of occupational disease epidemics. The limitations of traditional scientific approaches are explored and the notion that epidemics can be quantified and controlled through the straightforward application of scientific knowledge and tools is challenged. At the same time, the influence of power relationships and values on epidemiology is highlighted. The relative invisibility of occupational health epidemics and the low priority afforded to them are examined in relation to a number of factors including work and societal relations, workers' organisation, compensation arrangements and the role and status of occupational health professionals in relation to other groups. There is clearly a need to address the lack of political will to eliminate occupational disease epidemics that has characterised this field for many years. This chapter lays the ground for future strategies, arguing that these need to incorporate emerging models of social and lay epidemiology.

Introduction

Occupational hazards and risks can be removed, reduced or controlled depending upon technologies and policies available and adopted. However, identifying and dealing with occupational diseases is a complex and highly problematic process which is determined by social, cultural and political issues as well as scientific and medical knowledge and theories (Watterson, 1994a, b, c). Just as the more general definition of 'disease' is socially constructed, so too is that of occupational disease (Watterson, 1993; Dembe, 1996).

Occupational diseases may be either caused by or related to occupation and are endemic. However, the focus has usually been on occupationally caused diseases with the wider influences on occupational health ignored. It is difficult for instance to disentangle the aetiology and persistence of an asthma case in a worker who operates in a polluted workplace and lives in a polluted area nearby. Similar problems exist where there are multiple exposures to hazards: for instance when occupational stress and neurotoxins come together, disease incidence may rise. Too often work-related diseases are ignored, workers are not compensated and epidemics of such diseases go entirely unreported.

Early observers such as Agricola, Ramazzini and Potts all identified 'epidemics' 'of occupational diseases (Rantanen et al., 1994). However, the focus of historians on the plague and cholera may well have skewed our perception towards infectious diseases and away from occupational epidemics. Infectious diseases are feared by all, since they threaten higher socioeconomic groups by spreading out from areas of economic deprivation. In this context, diseases know no boundaries. Occupational disease epidemics on the other hand are usually 'ring fenced' and historically have affected mainly the lower socioeconomic groups. They are only rarely contagious and have historically been given less importance, often being left unchecked for centuries.

This does not mean that there has been no action on or campaigns about the 'old epidemics'. For instance, Arlidge, Legge and others highlighted the extent and damage from old industrial epidemics in the nineteenth century. Trade unions have sometimes pressed for action to remove occupational diseases and groups of workers have on occasions been the first to demand measures to end epidemics (Watterson, 1993, 1994a).

This chapter explores the ways in which occupational disease epidemics have been defined and constructed, the scale of these epidemics and the way they have been treated (or not) by health professionals. Two broad approaches to occupational disease prevention are analysed and a number of strategies for addressing epidemic occupational diseases are put forward.

Defining and constructing epidemics relevant to occupational health

Since 1960 the American Public Health Association's definition of an 'epidemic' has been widely adopted, centring on 'the occurrence in a community of a group of illnesses of similar nature, clearly in excess of normal expectation' (MacMahon *et al.*, 1960, p. 4). This definition replaced an earlier one which was restricted to acute outbreaks of infectious disease. Many categories of non-infectious occupational diseases qualify for 'epidemic' status within the APHA definition. Indeed, both the Finnish Institute of Occupational Health and the US National Institute for Occupational Safety and Health recognise occupational stress, occupational accidents, reproductive disorders and respiratory diseases in agriculture as occupational epidemics of the 1990s (Norppa and Haartz, 1992). Other conditions such as occupational cancers, musculoskeletal injuries, psychosocial stress and disorders and traumatic injuries are widely perceived as current research priorities (Rantanen, 1992, p. 6).

There may be 'old', 'new' and 'silent' epidemics. 'Old' epidemics are those which occurred decades ago and some consider are no longer with us. 'New' epidemics are those which have been identified relatively recently, while 'silent' epidemics are those where the diseases have existed for many decades but have not been recognised by medical or governmental agencies for recording and compensation purposes. Silent old epidemics may often become the 'new' epidemics. Until the mid-1990s, no occupational bronchitis was recognised in UK miners. Now that there are very few pits left open in the country and the numbers of miners have declined significantly, miners' bronchitis is recognised. Hence this new epidemic is really a silent epidemic stretching back over many decades. Many other new epidemics are in fact 'old' epidemics extending into new occupational groups and industries. In that 'endemic' diseases are those which occur frequently in a particular region or population, it is now clear that silent 'old' epidemics of occupational diseases are simply endemic diseases unrecognised.

New epidemics according to Finnish commentators include hanta viruses, musculoskeletal diseases, multiple chemical sensitivity, 'new' asthmatic and alveolar disorders and psychological conditions including burnout (Rantananen *et al.*, 1994). Yet the discovery of some of these is the result of increased attention to old and silent epidemics (Watterson, 1994c). A change in the social distribution of disease may serve to highlight hitherto neglected epidemics as may the exposure of new groups of workers to the old hazards and associated risks. For instance, effective action in response to some epidemics has often only occurred after economic and technical changes have resulted in increased exposure among the middle classes. Hence successful compensation claims for repetitive strain injuries increased when journalists and technical and scientific staff were affected alongside clerical and support staff as a consequence of increased computer use.

There are also epidemics that are recognised but are viewed by workers as part of the job, such as back pain for nurses and building workers, damaged knee joints for carpet layers and miners as well as colds and flu for teachers. In times of insecure or poor employment conditions these are likely to remain unchallenged. Job insecurity encourages employees not to disclose their occupational illnesses and recent research revealed that workers need to be healthier now than 20 years ago in order to keep their jobs (*Hazards* 58, 1997, p. 2).

Definitions of epidemics may vary between countries depending on differences in diagnosis and the interpretation of the significance of each disease. Budget limits set by governments for compensation also affect the definition of occupational disease epidemics, as can be demonstrated in relation to the epidemic of 'dementia' among Scandinavian painters but not among workers in other countries exposed to similar solvents. This variation is in part the result of different governments' responses to research evidence that occupational paint solvent exposures cause neurological damage.

There may be widely different burdens of proof used by societies to define diseases. In Ontario, Canada, the Occupational Diseases Panel uses a 'rebuttal presumption' approach where work factors are assumed to cause disease unless proved otherwise (*Hazards* 49, 1994, pp. 1–2). In other countries, such as the UK, it is generally assumed that work does not cause occupational illness unless an extensive body of research data is provided and a very high level of proof of causality established. Consequently, there seem to be relatively few occupational epidemics in the UK. At the same time, 'new' epidemics tend to be recognised at a more advanced stage and there are more 'silent' epidemics.

Paradoxically, large epidemics in the workplace may reflect good practice through effective reporting and recording of occupational diseases. A lack of epidemic records may indicate bad reporting and recording practice and not an absence of disease.

Rather than debating the nature of occupational disease epidemics, the problems of work-related ill health may be more effectively addressed by examining populations where exposure levels are at or above those levels known to cause disease. Concentration on 'sentinel events' is another way forward. In this context, sentinel events are those which provide early warning or a possible indication of occupational diseases otherwise missed by conventional epidemiological and toxicological methods. The use of sentinel events as a key concept in occupational health could redefine our understanding of epidemics to include reports by 'astute workers' and physicians (Hogstedt, 1994).

Supposedly neutral scientific debates are always influenced by issues of power and status and questions of occupational health are no exception. Hence, trade union and 'worker' definitions of epidemics may differ from those of 'experts' and professionals. In many cases, for example those of railway workers for fatigue, telegraphists for RSI, gas workers for bladder cancer, workers have identified epidemics long before health professionals have done so (Watterson, 1993).

The problem and size of occupational disease epidemics

Various problems exist in documenting accurately the precise causation and scale of occupational disease epidemics. For instance, workers may have multiple exposures to hazards or may move from job to job, therefore becoming untraceable for epidemiological studies and biological monitoring. This is the case with migrant agricultural workers in Africa, South America and the USA. There are similar problems for migrant industrial workers in the *maquiladoras* or with Mexican, Puerto Rican and Caribbean casual workers. Epidemics which occur may never be recorded in these circumstances.

Even where occupational diseases are recognised, they are significantly underreported. This is due to a variety of factors including lack of agreement between scientists, lack of resources and insufficient numbers of trained and informed occupational health staff. These problems are often underlined by a lack of political will to address work risks. Employers may be ignorant about their legal duties or reluctant to report diseases (O'Neill, 1995, pp. 105–6) while governments and insurance companies may also be unwilling to face up to the economic and social consequences of epidemics of occupational diseases.

Technologies which could be used to ascertain the extent of occupational diseases are in practice sometimes used instead to police the workforce. For example, the setting of tight standards for chemical exposures in the workplace has been resisted on the grounds that the technologies for monitoring very low level exposures have not existed. Recent developments in technology have allowed UK employers to use parts per billion technologies to measure traces of illegal drugs taken by their workforce outside work time (*Hazards* 55, 1996, pp. 8–9). Yet samples of lead, cadmium or arsenic – the causes of old epidemic diseases that are still with us – are rarely if at all measured to the nearest part per million.

Recognition of epidemics is also influenced by workers themselves, especially in the workplaces where trade unions are well organised. In such workplaces, effective health and safety action by workers at plant level may help to identify, define and measure occupational diseases better and so reduce and possibly prevent 'mini epidemics' (Watterson, 1994a). Similarly, in these workplaces epidemics may be better reported, compensation more systematically sought and efforts made to get diseases prescribed (Barth, 1982). In contrast, in unorganised or poorly organised workplaces and indeed unions, claims for prescribed industrial diseases are less likely to be made and many of the diseases are unlikely to be the focus of campaigns for recognition.

The impact of trade unions on 'marking up' and dealing with epidemics in the workplace is significant. In the UK, TUC-affiliated trade unions represent about a third of the workforce, yet they take about 70 per cent of all workplace personal injury cases. Organisations such as the Sheffield Occupational Health Project and Unemployed Centres, both of which have strong links with the unions, have revealed hitherto unreported or grossly underrecorded occupational epidemics in local populations including occupational deafness in Sheffield and mucous membrane disease in Sunderland (*Hazards* 46, 1994, p. 13; see also Pickvance, this volume). Here local expertise has identified hidden epidemics when national medical expertise has not. In one year, the Sheffield Occupational Health Project identified more cases of chrome ulceration in one small Sheffield factory than were recorded in all the official records for the entire country (*Hazards* 31, 1990, p. 40). In contrast, physicians have sometimes failed to recognise work-related diseases including epidemics of radiographers' asthma (O'Neill, 1995, p. 105) and hard metal disease (*Hazards* 20, 1988, pp. 6–7).

There is evidence that trade union-organised workplaces are healthier and safer than their unorganised counterparts (Watterson, 1994b; *Hazards* 58, 1997, p. 5). Trade unions may also play a role within the wider community, for example by representing employees in the common law setting and ensuring one form of recognition for epidemics, as has been the case with successful occupational stress claims. In the technical sphere, trade unions may challenge narrow definitions of prescribed industrial diseases as happened successfully with miners' obstructive airways disease. Coal miners have struggled against apathy and even hostility from medical and other professional groups in order to get pneumoconiosis and other respiratory diseases recognised. Finally, in society at large, trade unions may campaign to ensure that diseases such as RSI, stress and asthma are more widely known and subsequently legally or medically recognised. Medical research often catches up with workers' concerns decades after these have been voiced, gradually recognising new diseases flagged much earlier by employees (Barth, 1982; Weindling, 1985; Watterson, 1993).

Successful compensation claims are often taken as a basis for assessing the scale of occupational disease. Yet compensation systems contain many flaws which are extremely damaging to affected workers as well as often leading to underestimates of disease. Claimants continue to face difficulties in seeking benefits. Entitlement to legal support (*Hazards* 56, 1996, p. 7), the costs of court proceedings, the time taken to process legal claims, and the fairness of the legal system can all influence the number of successful compensation claims for occupational diseases. The protracted process of getting diseases prescribed sometimes means that, by the time this is done, the industries have moved on technologically or geographically. Hence only a small number of affected workers have been able to claim for the diseases they suffered; many having become ill and died before the right to claim was introduced. Late diagnosis of prescribed industrial diseases can have appalling direct consequences: for instance when UK miners' corpses were left for up to a fortnight in the front rooms of their houses because there were queues for postmortems to confirm the cause of death by industrial disease.

Miners' claims for pneumoconiosis and bronchitis also demonstrate the limitations of compensation systems where these rely on problematic medical evidence. Claims have been limited on the basis of percentage points of lung damage recorded by X-rays: above a certain level the disease has been accepted and compensated, below, it has not. These tests have meant the success of only one in eight applicants for compensation even though the tests could only identify restrictive and not obstructive lung disease (*Western Mail*, 7 April 1997).

Problems of occupational epidemic disease recognition have been further compounded by the failure of academic and scientific research to address the subject. Hunter's classic *Diseases of Occupations* refers only to one epidemic, the apparently mouse-borne virus of keratocon-junctivitis in US shipyard workers during 1941 (Hunter, 1975, p. 96). This reluctance to write about 'epidemics' of occupational disease has continued into recent decades and in the indexes of the *British Journal of Industrial Medicine* up until the time of writing there is just one reference to epidemics. This came in 1951 with reference to epidemic influenza in industry: an illustration of the importance given to infectious diseases in epidemic history. Generally, it is an exception rather than the rule to find occupational or environmental epidemics described in the medical and scientific literature (Epstein, 1978; Navarro and Berman, 1983; Weindling, 1985; Buck *et al.*, 1988, pp. 67, 415–51; Weekes *et al.*, 1991, p. 377).

However, this only partially explains the gaps in information about the scale of occupational health problems. In addition to the lack of epidemiological research on occupational health (Hunter, 1975, p. 96), a low status has been accorded to occupational health researchers and practitioners, especially to occupational hygienists, engineers and others who may often hold the key to preventing disease.

There has been a mismatch between the way in which public health practitioners respond to infectious disease epidemics and how those in occupational medicine respond to similar developments (Schilling, 1981, p. 6; Bres, 1986, p. 3). This relates in part to a greater public concern about infectious diseases than about non-infectious occupational diseases. Moreover, those creating occupational hazards have often been the very same people who are supplying the data and sitting on or influencing those bodies which prescribe new diseases. Their wish not to pay out civil compensation and high insurance premiums and also to avoid criminal prosecution for the morbidity and mortality of employees from occupational diseases also plays a part in explaining inaction in relation to occupational epidemics. As a result the financial costs of these problems have historically been borne by victims, their families and communities and the tax payer.

The role of occupational medicine and related disciplines has been significant in limiting identification and recognition of occupational epidemics. These disciplines have proved to be remarkably self-effacing. They have often stressed low hazards, low risks and counselled against overestimating diseases which are occupationally caused or related. The reasons for this are complex. Occupational health practitioners are, unusually, often employed directly by industries, public organisations and others and hence their livelihoods can depend very directly on their employer. This can lead to implicit or explicit pressure to downplay or suppress reports and research identifying occupational disease epidemics (see Epstein, 1978; Ives, 1985). Occupational health professionals may also work within a personnel structure in which concerns such as resource management and day to day industrial relations are given greater priority than occupational diseases.

In the industrial countries where the discipline has been most developed, occupational medicine has remained conservative in advocating precautionary policies despite evidence of workplace disease epidemics (Watterson, 1993, 1995). This conservatism may be the result of an overemphasis on the value of negative or cautious epidemiology by those working in the discipline seeking to establish greater clinical and scientific credibility. This caution could well lead to an underreporting or downplaying of work-caused epidemics.

Despite the problems of measuring occupational disease epidemics, there is substantial evidence of epidemic occupational diseases (International Agency for Research on Cancer, 1995, pp. 194, 336; National Toxicity Programme, 1994). Data suggest that these epidemics have swept the world for many decades often unchecked. In 1995, the WHO estimated that cases of occupational diseases affected between 37 and 84 cases per 10,000 among the global workforce. This provides occupational disease figures of between 7,920,000 and 18,050,000 out of a workforce of 2,150,000,000: truly a global epidemic (Mikheev, 1994, pp. 30–1).

In Europe, researchers have recently analysed self-reported data from 15,500 workers in fifteen EU member states, revealing occupational diseases on an epidemic scale (Paoli et al., 1996). In the USA in 1978 the National Institute of Environmental Health Sciences estimated that one in five cancers was linked to occupation. In the UK at the same time, one commentator predicted that asbestos exposures would kill more people in Britain than were killed in the armed forces during the Second World War; an estimate which represented a preventable 'epidemic of asbestos-related diseases' (Dalton, 1979, p. 7). Occupational diseases in the USA and Europe during the 1980s can only be interpreted as of epidemic proportions (Elling, 1986). Likewise epidemiological and toxicological studies have identified epidemics of illnesses among workers and communities affected by industrial pollutants and chemicals such as dioxins and PCBs which have been in workplaces for many decades (Gibbs, 1995). In Bulgaria, 30,000 workers are exposed to lead and about 70 per cent of plants surveyed in 1990 had lead levels above 0.05mg/m^3 (WHO, 1995, p. 405).

Finland has some of the best occupational health disease prevention policies in the world as well as one of the finest occupational disease reporting systems. Yet the figures suggest that even in Finland the scale of the occupational disease epidemic is enormous. These are effectively old epidemics caused by chemicals and dust hazards which have been in use for decades if not centuries including epoxy resins, cobalt, isocyanates, asbestos, chromium, nickel, formaldehyde, organic solvents, bioaerosols, lead mercury, wood dust, halogenated hydrocarbons, styrene, mineral fibres, aldehydes, cadmium and flour and grain dusts (Antilla, 1992). If this is the size of the old epidemic problem in Finland, it is certain to be far worse elsewhere in Europe where identification and recording systems and occupational hygiene controls are often inferior.

Epidemics of occupational disease may vary significantly in size and impact. On the one hand, they may be relatively small but have a very large impact on the individuals involved, as in the case of angiosarcoma due to exposure to vinyl chloride and bladder and lung cancer in industrial societies. On the other hand, they may be widespread as in the case of pesticide poisonings which affect approximately 3 million people each year, with the bulk of these in developing countries (Jeyaratnam, 1995, p. 152).

Table 6.1 European Foundation 1996 Survey of EU working conditions

Disease or exposure	Percentage of workforce affected (total = 147,000)
Occupational back injuries	30
Occupational stress	28
Heavy load work	33
Noise	28
Repetitive movements (hand/arm)	57

Source: Paoli et al., 1996

Table 6.2 Workers in WHO European Region facing significant risks of epidemic occupational disease

Likely epidemic disease	Exposure	Percentage or number of workforce exposed
Occupational deafness	80–85dB	15–50%
Vibration – tools	1–80% of exposed workers have signs of damage	Up to 5%
Vibration – vehicles	Whole body vibration	5–10% of workforce
Fibrogenic dusts (Poland)		200,000
Harmful substances (Poland)		130,000

Source: WHO, 1995

Table 6.3   Causes of occupational asthma epidemics by industry or occupation

Industry/occupation	Some long established asthma causes
Health services	Formaldehyde, glutaraldehyde, penicillin, latex
Construction	Mineral fibre, epoxy resins, isocyanates, asphalt and diesel fumes, cement and plaster board, zinc, woods, welding fumes
Engineering	Nickel, chrome, vanadium, foundry resins, soldering fumes, degreasing chemicals. Stainless steel and other welding

Source: O'Neill, 1995

Table 6.4   Percentage of occupational diseases caused by chemicals

Country	Percentage of workforce affected
Finland	up to 41.6%
Germany	56%
Hungary	28%
Poland	29.5%

Source: WHO, 1995

The scale of the European epidemics in the 1990s is confirmed by Tables 6.1–6.4. These tables illustrate the fact that exposures to old hazards such as noise, vibration, toxic dusts and chemicals continue to exact a heavy toll at the same time as the introduction of new materials and risks is contributing to epidemic diseases. The European survey described in Table 6.1 further found that workers on fixed-term or temporary contracts faced the worst hazards. Hence epidemics of occupational disease continue to disproportionately affect the most economically vulnerable groups.

Underpinning policies influencing definition, recording and treatment of occupational disease epidemics

There are two broad approaches to occupational disease. First, the 'scientific', which in its least effective manifestation appears as scientism, and which Costanza and Cornwell (1992) have termed the 'technological optimist' approach. It is based on the assumption that science

Table 6.5   Two models of occupational health policy

1 Scientism/expertist model	– based on scientific certainty or 'beyond reasonable doubt' – scientific solutions always exist to any problem – technological optimists – no need for laws or openness as the experts know what they are doing but no one else does – no public access to information – undemocratic and unaccountable
2 Socioparticipative model	– based on participative model of health care and health promotion not the medical model – based on freedom of information provisions which are funded to work effectively – toxics use registers – uses lay epidemiology and intuitive toxicology as well as conventional science and is non-jargonistic – risk mapping – 'prudent avoidance' – prudent pessimists following 'balance of probabilities' assessment – occupational health preventive approach based on absence of evidence not being the same as evidence of absence – incorporating clean production and toxics reduction on chemical hazards – Italy in parts in 1980s, USA in part in 1970s based on Danish and Swedish examples of good practice

Source: Based on Bagnara, 1985, adapted by Watterson, 1994

can remove or effectively control any occupational hazard or risk created by any technology, ensuring high safety margins. Its advocates adopt the 'beyond reasonable doubt' level of proof used by lawyers. Hence, they insist on the establishment of proof that hazards exist and that high risks are attached to materials and processes before any precautionary actions are taken (Costanza and Cornwell, 1992). Drawing on scientific methods, this approach often involves a testing of the null hypothesis: the onus is on the public and community to prove the danger rather than the scientific investigator to demonstrate safety.

In this system a high level of predictive power is assumed and the scientific method itself is seen as almost foolproof. However, our ability to assess and predict occupational health risks over the long term is in fact limited (MarkSmith and Christiani, 1994). Even hazards such as carcinogenicity and reproductive risks associated with lead are poorly understood. The introduction of lead into petrol and the development of CFCs for commercial use were considered by technological optimists as presenting no problems at the time. It is now known that these actions led to widespread lead contamination of working and wider environments, contributing to an epidemic of skin cancers due to damage to the ozone layer. Hence prudent avoidance rather than endless or often repeated risk assessments appears to be the way forward (*Workers' Health International Newsletter* 49/50, 1997, p. 29).

The asbestos story is perhaps the most salutary one for the technological optimists. It reveals underplaying and underreporting over centuries of the principal occupational disease epidemic in the world. The initial assumption that all forms of asbestos were safe gave way to the insistence that some forms of asbestos were safe and then that

Table 6.6   Dates of UK knowledge on asbestos

First century AD	Pliny notes slaves working in asbestos mines die young from lung disease
1857	Asbestos products appear in England
1898	Her Majesty's Factory Inspectorate note evil effects of asbestos fibres
1906	Dr Murray in UK diagnoses death of a worker from asbestos disease
1929	Leeds coroner calls for public enquiry after death of asbestos worker
1930	Merewether and Price in UK report epidemic of asbestos disease in UK workers
1955	Doll produces report on lung cancer deaths which convinces scientists 20 years after high levels of lung cancer in asbestos workers was reported
1970	1969 Asbestos Regulations introduced
1982	Peto predicts about 50,000 asbestos-induced deaths in UK. Critics state it is a gross underestimate
1995	HSE sharply revises upwards its estimates of asbestos-related deaths for 1995–2025

Source: London Hazards Centre, 1995

some exposures to asbestos were safe. The dangers of asbestos have continued to be underestimated as Table 6.6 illustrates.

Geoffrey Rose observed that 'have not noticed is not the same as does not exist' (Rose, 1991). One governmental or workplace coping strategy for occupational disease epidemics is not to look for or notice them: if it can be argued that they do not exist then there is no need for action. Rose also noted that large numbers of people exposed to low level contamination over a long period of time may represent a greater public health (and in this case occupational health) hazard than small numbers of workers exposed to high levels of contamination over short periods of time (Rose, 1992). Yet this approach to occupational disease epidemics appears to have been lost sight of in the 1990s. We tend to focus on immediate or shorter term threats to health because of their apparent urgency. These often relate to infectious conditions such as TB and HIV which manifest themselves quite quickly. Epidemic diseases which develop over a longer period such as hepatitis C, respiratory diseases and immune system damage are in contrast initially less visible, life threatening or dramatic.

The opposite to the scientist/scientism model is the 'socioparticipative model' which recognises from the outset that science has limits. The model tends to be more democratic and open on questions of decision making and less expertist. It works along what Costanza has termed the 'prudent pessimist' line, building in greater safety margins and drawing on the legal concept of the balance of probabilities (Watterson, 1982) which errs in favour of exposed workers and communities in the assessment of risk. This approach also questions who benefits from technological innovation and recognises the significance of data gaps and conflicting models of mechanisms of toxicity, as in relation to chemicals or dose/response/damage relationships in exposures to physical hazards such as low level radiation, electromagnetic fields, noise, cold, heat, vibration and humidity.

The socioparticipative model is essentially geared to preventing occupational disease and hence avoiding occupational epidemics. It does not depend on what in a practical sense is a futile discussion about disease and then epidemic definition. It emphasises 'the healthy and safe workplace' rather than the 'healthy and safe worker', with the balance of probabilities always operating in favour of the employee who might be exposed to known or unknown hazards. Hence epidemics are dealt with by avoiding exposure. It is not a Utopian approach, however, as it is informed by science and builds on cumulative research identifying the flaws of previous risk assessments.

Why are old epidemics still with us?

The reasons for old epidemic persistence are numerous and may vary between places, companies, industry and countries. However, several reasons may have general applicability and validity. Least convincing are suggestions that the lack of data about a disease leads to an inability to identify it or address its causes. Many occupational diseases such as cancers were identified a long time ago: coal soot in 1775, bitumen coal tar in 1876, coal tar fumes in 1936, shale paraffin oil in 1876 and petroleum paraffin oil in 1910, lubricating oils in 1910 and 1930, creosote in 1920, benzene in 1928, arsenic in 1822, nickel in 1932 and chromates in 1935 (Hubert, cited in Barth, 1982, p. 7). It was certainly not a lack of data which explained inaction.

In addition to the lack of data, inadequate methodologies for the identification of epidemics are often cited as a reason for the failure of effective prevention. Today this relates to causal and random clusters in specific industries where it is suggested that the numbers of exposed workers are too small to allow for identification which meets established statistical criteria and standards on epidemics. Yet recent events such as the BSE crisis demonstrate that it is not always possible simply to prove or disprove a connection between excesses of disease and an occupational or environmental factor. This does not amount to an argument for inaction, and stronger actions could have been taken to prevent these workplace disease epidemics (Watterson, 1994c).

Negative epidemiology relates to studies which are not capable of disproving a link between an exposure and a disease but are sometimes presented or interpreted as doing so. Such studies may be poorly designed and insensitive to certain diseases, too small to produce meaningful results or contain other flaws such as the use of invalid control groups, inaccurate exposure data, incorrect categorisation of exposed and non-exposed workers, failure to register exposure levels or measure such levels over a sufficiently long period, random errors and crude or irrelevant morbidity indicators (Hernberg, 1992). The problems have been compounded by often long latency periods in the development of occupational diseases and the fact that technologies move on and leave affected workers behind (Gee, in Doyal *et al.*, 1983).

These factors, together with the lack of enforcement officers and the failure to enforce occupational health laws are likely to ensure the continuation of 'old epidemics'. The same could be said of the lack of information and advice on how to avoid these diseases and the existence of a legal system which limits workers' chances of receiving compensation while failing to penalise employers who create 'old' epidemics. On the other hand, a greater likelihood of compensation, more cases going through the courts, higher awards for victims and bigger insurance premiums for offenders would all help to cut occupational disease rates.

Factory production systems in industrial societies can create conditions in which occupational disease epidemics flourish (Burawoy, 1985). For example, 'new management techniques' involving continuous improvement methods, sub-contracting, delayering and teamworking present threats of psychological and physiological work related disease (Pickvance, 1997; Richardson, 1997; see also Daykin, this volume). Such techniques are of course not new, the problems created by casualisation including the use of 'gangmasters' and gangs in agriculture as well as lump labour in the construction industry and in the docks and have long been documented. These problems include poor workplace organisation, poor health and safety management, anti-trade unionism, low levels of occupational health knowledge, deficient equipment and materials and poor training, supervision and information to employees. In some western European countries there has been a move back to 'sweatshop' economies and homeworking. As well as the creation of new epidemics this may lead to a resurgence of old ones if workers are exposed to hazards such as solvent and pesticides exposure without the controls which may have previously existed in large factories.

There is a widely held assumption that new technology removes old hazards and epidemics, going on to create new ones. This is only a partial picture. Many old epidemics continue because of the persistence of some hazards and traditional processes, such as asbestos and lead, in or around workplaces. It is often cheaper to leave these materials and processes rather than remove them and as a consequence new and old epidemics may occur side by side. For example, within the microelectronics industry many new technologies have been introduced at the same time as old solvents and other hazards remain.

New technologies may well bring new risks but this is not inevitable and can be avoided by careful consideration of the human element. However, this rarely happens. Hence new technologies can create major new workplace epidemics as well as exacerbating old ones. For example, prior to the widespread introduction of display screen equipment people with less than perfect eyesight would have been able to perform many workplace tasks. This technology now causes problems for people with even minor eye defects and, for the rest of us, 'computer vision syndrome' (*Hazards* 58, 1997, pp. 8–9).

Ways forward

Responses to epidemics should build on careful understanding of the aetiology of each disease and the adoption of the public health precautionary approach, which itself relies on valid observations about the nature and location of each outbreak. Together with the 'prudent pessimist' philosophy this approach seems most likely to succeed in curtailing old epidemics and preventing new ones. Its emphasis is far less on defining occupational diseases and far more on identifying hazards and ensuring their removal or control.

Some countries, such as Finland, map occupational risks rather than outcomes in the form of occupational diseases. This allows risk reduction strategies to be applied while the hazard is still present. Other countries, such as the UK, rely on tracking outcomes, hence risk reduction measures are often only applied after workers' health has been damaged and sometimes when the technology causing the problem has moved on.

Old epidemics need to be controlled by clear regulations setting minimum standards and, when dealing with substances such as carcinogens, teratogens and respiratory sensitisers, perhaps bans or very rigid engineering controls. Since information *per se* does not prevent occupational disease, such regulations need to be underpinned by effective information, proper advice and meaningful enforcement and fines (Miettinen, 1995, pp. 116–18).

Finally, the regulation of occupational hazards in one country should not allow for their export to another. There are many examples of hazardous industries, processes and materials being exported from industrial nations to developing countries where their impact is even greater because of double standards or weaker controls (Castleman, 1985). These problems are likely to be compounded by recent developments including the deregulation of health and safety, the growth of child labour and the development of sweatshop economies (Jeyaratnam, 1992; Pearce *et al.*, 1994). Old epidemics such as silicosis and mesothelioma seem likely to increase in certain regions such as South Africa where the burden of disease and disability among some groups is already high.

The physician, pathologist and social epidemiologist, Rudolf Virchow observed in the nineteenth century that medicine was a social science and politics was nothing more than medicine on a grand scale (Rosen, 1974, pp. 61–7). Tackling epidemics of occupational disease in this context is a political and economic process and not merely a scientific one. Hence attacks on continuing 'old' epidemics should be informed by participatory research and worker epidemiology. Clusters of disease reported by 'astute' workers and physicians should be followed up as carefully as the results of experimental research (Hogstedt, 1994, p. 17). By adopting the prudent pessimist approach and using sentinel events about likely incidents and clusters of occupational disease, occupational diseases may be tackled effectively at source rather than after adverse health outcomes have been documented in 'epidemic reports'.

These strategies and tactics are not inimical to sustainable economic growth in any society. The Toxics Use Reduction Institute in Massachusetts has provided evidence that policies on cleaner production and toxics reduction, as well as effective ergonomic design, meaningful work organisation and empowerment, can improve productivity, quality and efficiency as well as environmental standards (*Workers' Health International Newsletter* 49/50, 1997, pp. 28–9). Recruitment and retention of staff is also likely to be enhanced in workplaces where the risk of occupational disease is minimised. Hence, where society pays the full costs of epidemic occupational diseases, prevention is undoubtedly a major source of social and economic benefit.

Acknowledgements

I am grateful to Rory O'Neill, David Gee and the editors for constructive comments on a draft of this paper and to Leslie London and Simon Pickvance for providing much useful information.

References

Antilla, A. (1992) *Occupational Chemical Exposure in Finland*. Helsinki: Finnish Institute of Occupational Health.

Bagnara, S., Misit, R. and Wintersberger, H. (eds) (1985) *Work and Health in the 1980s*. Berlin: Sigma.

Barth, P.S. (with Hunt, H.A.) (1982) *Workers' Compensation and Work-related Illnesses and Diseases*. Cambridge, MA: MIT.

Bres, P. (1986) *Public Health Action in Emergencies caused by Epidemics*. Geneva: WHO.

British Journal of Industrial Medicine, Vol. 1–end, 1940s–1990s.

Buck, C., Llopis, A., Najera, E. and Terris, M. (1988) *The Challenge of Epidemiology: Issues and Selected Readings*. Scientific Publications No. 505. Washington: Pan American Health Organisation.

Burawoy, M. (1985) *The Politics of Production: Factory Regimes under Capitalism and Socialism*. London: Verso.

Castleman, B. (1985) 'The double standard in industrial hazards' in J.H. Ives (ed.), *The Export of Hazard: Transnational Corporations and Environmental Control Issues*. London: Routledge & Kegan Paul.

Costanza, R. and Cornwell, L. (1992) 'The 4P approach to dealing with scientific uncertainty', *Environment*, **34**.

Dalton, A. (1979) *Asbestos: Killer Dust*. London: BSSRS.

Dembe, A.E. (1996) *Occupation and Disease: How Social Factors Affect the Conception of Work-related Disorders*. New Haven, CT: Yale University Press.

Doyal, L., Green, K. and Irwin, I. (1983) *Cancer in Britain: The Politics of Prevention*. London: Pluto.

Elling, R.H. (1986) *The Struggle for Workers' Health*. New York: Baywood.

Epstein, S. (1978) *The Politics of Cancer*. San Francisco: Sierra Club Books.

Gibbs, L.M. (ed.) (1995) *Dying from Dioxin*. Boston: South End Press.

Hazards (1988) No. 20: 6–7; (1990) No. 31: 40; (1994) No. 46: 13; No. 49: 1–2; (1996) No. 55: 8–9; No. 56: 7; (1997) No. 58: 2, 5, 8–9.

Hernberg, S. (1992) *Introduction to Occupational Epidemiology*. Clesea, MI: Lewis.

Hogstedt, C. (1994) 'From sentinel observations to practical actions', in J. Rantanen, S. Lehtinen, R. Kalim, *et al*.: 17–26.

Hunter, D. (1975) *Diseases of Occupations*. 5th edn. London: Hodder & Stoughton.

International Agency for Research on Cancer (1995) *Wood Dust and Formaldehyde*, Monograph Volume 62. Lyons: International Agency for Research on Cancer.

Ives, J.H. (ed.) (1985) *The Export of Hazard: Transnational Corporations and Environmental Control Issues*. London: Routledge & Kegan Paul.

Jeyaratnam, J. (ed.) (1992) *Occupational Health in Developing Countries*. Oxford: Oxford University Press.

Jeyaratnam, J. (1995) 'Research to policy decisions' in J. Rantanen, S. Lehtinen, R. Kalim, *et al*.

London Hazards Centre (1995) *The Asbestos Hazards Handbook*. London: London Hazards Centre Trust.

MacMahon, B., Pugh, T.F. and Ipsen, J. (1960) *Epidemiologic Methods*. London: J.A. Churchill.

Marksmith, C., Christiani, D.C. and Kelsey, K.T. (eds) (1994) *Chemical Risk Assessment and Occupational Health*. Westport, CT: Auburn House.

Miettinen, O.S. (1995) 'Managing occupational and environmental health hazards: health and economic outcomes', in J. Rantanen, S. Lehtinen, R. Kalim, *et al*.

Mikheev, M. (1994) 'New epidemics – the challenge for international health work' in J. Rantanen.

National Toxicity Program (1994) *Seventh Annual Report on Carcinogens*. Washington: NTP/NIH/NCI/NIEHS/FDA/CDC.

Navarro, V. and Berman, D.M. (eds) (1983) *Health and Work under Capitalism*. New York: Baywood.

Norppa, H. and Haartz, J.C. (eds) (1992) 'Occupational epidemics in the 1990s', *Scand. J. Work Environment and Health*, **18**(2) 136.

O'Neill, R. (1995) *Asthma at Work*. Sheffield: TUC/Sheffield Occupational Health Project.

Paoli, P. (1996) *Second European Survey on Working Conditions 1996*. Data set. Dublin: European Foundation for the Improvement of Living and Working Conditions.

Pearce, N., Matos, E., Vainio, H., Boffetta, P. and Kogevinas, M. (eds) (1994) *Occupational Cancer in Developing Countries*. Lyons: International Agency for Research on Cancer.

Pickvance, S. (1997) *Taking Control at Work*. *Hazards* 58: 3–5.

Rantanen, J. (1992) 'Priority setting and evaluation as tools for planning research strategies' in H. Norppa and J.C. Haartz (eds), *Occupational Epidemics in the 1990s. Scand. J. Work Environment and Health*, **18**(2): 5–7.

Rantanen, J., Lehtinen, S., Kalimo, R. *et al.* (eds) (1994) *New Epidemics in Occupational Health*. Helsinki: Finnish Institute of Occupational Health.

Rantanen, J., Lehtinen, S., Hernberg, S. *et al.* (eds) (1995) *From Research to Prevention: Managing Occupational and Environmental Health Hazards*. People and Work Research Report No. 4. Helsinki: Finnish Institute of Occupational Health.

Richardson, C. (1997) *Tricks and Traps*. Technology and Work Programme. Lowell: University of Massachusetts.

Rose, G. (1991) 'Environmental health: problems and perspectives', *Journal of the Royal College of Physicians*, **25**: 48–52.

Rose, G. (1992) *The Strategy of Preventive Medicine*. Oxford: Oxford Medical Publications.

Rosen, G. (1974) *From Medical Police to Social Police: Essays on the History of Health Care*. New York: Science History Publications.

Schilling, R.S.F (ed.) (1981) *Occupational Health Practice*. London: Butterworth.

Vainio, H. (1997) 'Lead and cancer – association or causation?', *Scand. J. Work, Environment and Health*, **23**: 1–3.

Watterson, A.E. (1982) More effective control of pesticides. *Occupational Health*, **34**: 409–14.

Watterson, A.E. (1993) 'Occupational health in the gas industry' in Platt, S., Thomas, H., Scott, S. and Williams, G.

Watterson, A.E. (1994a) 'Whither lay epidemiology in occupational and environmental health?', *Journal of Public Health Medicine*, **16**: 270–4.

Watterson, A.E. (1994b) 'British and related European workplace health and safety policies: no major changes likely', *New Solutions: Journal of Environmental and Occupational Health Policy*, **5**: 62–71.

Watterson, A.E. (1994c) 'International attitudes to organophosphates', *Farmers' Ill-Health and OP Sheepdips*. Proceedings of the Conference held on 26 March 1994 at Plymouth Postgraduate Medical School, Plymouth, UK.

Watterson, A.E. (1995) *Breast Cancer and the Links with Environmental and Occupational Carcinogens: Public Health Dilemmas and Policies*. Leicester: Centre for Occupational and Environmental Health.

Weekes, J.L., Levy, B.S. and Wagner, G.R. (eds) (1991) *Preventing Occupational Disease and Injury*. Washington: APHA.

Weindling, P. (ed.) (1985) *The Social History of Occupational Health*. London: Croom Helm.

WHO European Centre for Environment and Health (1995) *Concern for Europe's Tomorrow: Health and the Environment in the WHO European Region*. Stuttgart: Wissenschaftliche Verlagsgesellschaft mbH.

Workers' Health International Newsletter (1997) No. 49/50: 28–29.

7 TRACKING THE INVISIBLE: SCIENTIFIC INDICATORS OF THE HEALTH HAZARDS IN WOMEN'S WORK

Karen Messing

The critique of bias in occupational epidemiology continues with this chapter, which demonstrates that most research and practice in the field of occupational health and safety has been insensitive to specifically female concerns. This bias needs to be challenged by the reorientation of research priorities and by the development of new methods that take both biological and social differences between men and women into account. Drawing mainly on examples from studies carried out in collaboration with trades unions in Quebec, this chapter outlines the changes needed to develop gender-sensitive practice in occupational health research. It demonstrates the need for the use of more appropriate indicators for monitoring work-related damage, for the elimination of methodological techniques such as 'adjusting for sex' and for changes in government policies on issues such as compensation. Above all, it stresses the importance of placing women's occupational health concerns within the broader framework of their daily lives.

Introduction

I was recently asked to give a talk for Women's Health Day at a medical school. When I asked the colleague who contacted me what she wanted

127

me to talk about, she said that she had heard I could talk about women's occupational health. 'But,' she said hesitantly, 'I have no idea what that is.' It is a little puzzling that such a statement could be made by a biology professor interested in women's health, some twenty years after the publication of Jeanne Stellman's *Women's Work, Women's Health* (1978). But it did not surprise me. There is still very little cross-fertilization between specialists in women's health and those in occupational health. It is still hard to find information about occupational effects on such women's health problems as osteoporosis, age at menopause and breast cancer, although some work on the last subject is emerging (Pukkala *et al.*, 1995; Goldberg and Labrèche, 1996). Chemical exposures of laboratory technicians, cleaners and hairdressers have been little studied, and the same is true for musculoskeletal risks of women's jobs in factories and services (Guo *et al.*, 1995).

Although researchers are starting to produce information on health problems in some women's jobs (Messing *et al.*, 1995; Messing, 1998) the knowledge is not yet at the fingertips of policy makers. In my own province of Quebec, Canada, the policy manual of the Ministry of Health and Social Services (1992) speaks of the occupational causes of musculoskeletal (pp. 86–87) and of psychological (p. 109) problems, notes elsewhere that women have more of these problems, but never makes the connection with women's working conditions (Ministère de la santé et des services sociaux du Quebec, 1992). Although the strategies for health promotion proposed on pages 131–183 include steps toward economic and social equality for women, none of the prevention strategies makes any mention of women's work as a source of their health risks, and the occupational health risks mentioned are in male-dominated sectors such as forestry, metallurgy and construction.

Many specialists think that the lack of interest in women's occupational health is normal and not a problem. They reason that women's jobs are relatively easy and safe. Women are often excluded from obviously demanding and dangerous jobs, and their health is therefore relatively well protected in the workplace. Also, jobs are a relatively minor aspect of women's lives. Thus, these scientists see no particular need to pay attention to women's working conditions from a health and safety standpoint. On those rare occasions when there could be a problem, they suppose that women will be included in the examination of health problems in mixed occupations. After all, women's reproductive health is quite well studied (Filkins and Kerr, 1993) and it is well known that being employed has a beneficial effect on women's health (Doyal, 1995, pp. 152–5).

If we believe in the foregoing principles, we will indeed see no need to study women's occupational health. In this chapter I would like to present an alternative view. I think that women's occupational health problems are relatively invisible to scientists because they are using inappropriate methods. The theory and practice of research in occupational health developed at a time when there were relatively few paid women workers. Women and men have very different jobs and responsibilities, so that the health risks in women's jobs may not emerge from a study of men's jobs (Armstrong and Armstrong, 1993). Most concepts and methods in use in the field have developed in relation to jobs usually held by men, to male physiology and to male-pattern lifestyles. Given this bias, it is not surprising that health problems related to women's bodies, jobs and family responsibilities are misunderstood and underestimated. Even the research in reproductive health has usually been limited to foetal problems such as spontaneous abortions, low birthweight and malformation, without discussion of the effects of working conditions on the women themselves.

The consequences of this ignorance and underestimation are very serious. They can be expressed as two vicious circles (Figures 7.1 and 7.2). Figure 7.1 shows the circle relating to research. We can take occupational cancer as an example of a scientific field where women's problems are understudied. Zahm and her colleagues (1994) found that, of 1233 studies of occupational cancer published in major scien-

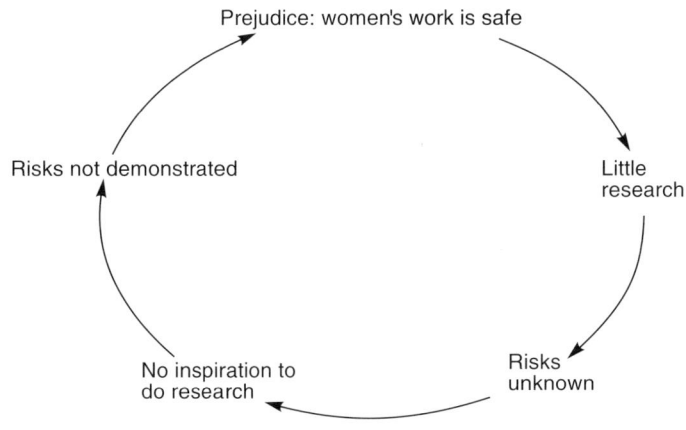

Figure 7.1   The vicious circle in scientific research on women's occupational health

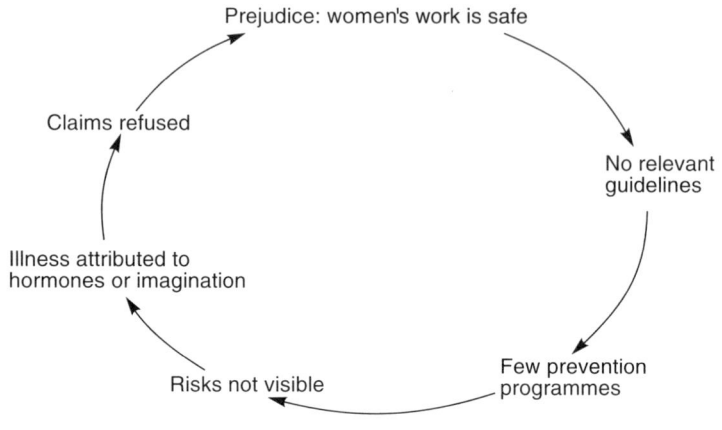

Figure 7.2   The vicious circle in prevention activities in jobs
held by women

tific journals in the 1980s and 1990s, only 14 per cent analysed data concerning women workers. On the basis of this lack of information, women have then been excluded from major studies on the grounds that they do not get occupational cancers and that it would be a waste of money to include them (Messing, 1994). Thus, the exclusion of women from scientific studies has created a circular situation where there is evidence of health problems only among men, leading to a reluctance to study women because of an impression that not many women get occupational disease.

The second vicious circle, involving ignorance of women's occupational diseases, concerns intervention. Because of the prejudice that women's work is safe, there are few prevention programmes in jobs where women are employed in services and factories. Thus, hazards are not discovered and standards are not developed for these jobs. When women experience health problems related to their jobs, they cannot claim for compensation based on known risk factors. Their allegations are not supported by those charged with improving health and safety (Lippel, in press). Instead, their problems are attributed to personal weaknesses, psychological difficulties or imagination. There is little pressure to improve the situation.

In Quebec for example, priorities for intervention in occupational health and safety have been set by employment sector (Messing and

Boutin, 1997). The economy is divided into six sectors, ranging from construction and chemicals (Sector 1) to health services, teaching and insurance (Sector 6). The Quebec Occupational Health and Safety Commission has set regulations for the first two sectors, requiring that employers prepare prevention programmes, pay employee representatives to do prevention work and form joint employer–employee prevention committees. These two sectors include only 5 per cent of all women workers (but a third of male workers). In the third sector, employers must prepare a prevention programme but need not provide the other supports for prevention activities. These first three sectors, including only 15 per cent of women workers, have more than eight times the number of inspections as the bottom three sectors (Commission de la santé et de la sécurité du travail du Québec, 1993, Tables 68 and 77). We can see from these numbers that the work that women do is not considered dangerous and that this perception has important implications for prevention. In the rest of the chapter I will show: first, that the indicators used to assess the health effects of employment do not work very well for the jobs usually held by women; second, that some research practices used to assess occupational hazards hide the risks in women's jobs; and third, that it is possible to use other methods to reveal these hidden risks.

Indicators of health effects of women's jobs

The priorities for intervention in Quebec were established primarily on the basis of statistics on work accidents. Those sectors with the highest numbers of accidents were, by and large, given the highest priority. It is therefore inevitable that sectors with large numbers of women would be allocated a low priority since women in Quebec have many fewer work accidents than men, as is true of other jurisdictions (Robinson, 1989; Laurin, 1991).

However, when we look at industrial disease, we see a somewhat different picture (Table 7.1). Women workers have more industrial diseases than men (Messing and Boutin, 1997). In other words, while men are concentrated in sectors where there is a risk of accidents, women work in areas where the dangers are less obvious, where health damage builds up over time.

Women are still not compensated very often because there are more than ten recognized work accidents in Quebec for one case of recognised industrial disease. This is no doubt because, even though work accidents are often contested, it is much easier to establish that a work

Table 7.1   Gender ratios in recognised work accidents and industrial
diseases, Quebec, 1992

	Recognised work accidents/100 workers			Recognised industrial diseases/1000 workers		
	F	M	F M	F	M	F M
All sectors	2.12	5.52	0.38	1.38	1.04	1.33

accident has occurred and that the worker's health damage is related
to the accident. If a construction worker has fallen off a scaffolding
and broken his leg, the damage is immediately visible and there is not
much question that it occurred at work.

Since industrial diseases build up over time, the link to the workplace is harder to make. The worker makes the same movement thousands of times a day and her elbow begins to hurt. After several years
she may get an epicondylitis that prevents her from doing that movement. When this happens, she or her doctor may possibly relate the
elbow joint inflammation to her job, but often they do not make the
connection. She may attribute the pain to the time she bumped her
elbow on the cupboard door while making supper, or to carrying heavy
grocery bags. Faced with pain at work, she may change jobs or leave
the workplace, so that her epicondylitis will never be picked up by a
scientist studying her former workplace.

Therefore, we need indicators that will allow us to see the damage
caused by the kinds of jobs women do. One such indicator, sickness
absence, has been proposed by several researchers in North America
and in Europe (Bourbonnais *et al.*, 1992; Alexanderson, 1998). Chevalier *et al.* (1987) used sickness absence to show that certain working
conditions at a French gas and electric company were associated with
absence. Bourbonnais and colleagues (1992) found that sickness
absence with a medical certificate was related to working conditions
among nurses.

The use of this indicator to assess the risks of women's working
conditions poses several problems, some of which may involve gender
insensitivity on the part of the investigators (Brooke and Price, 1989;
Deguire and Messing, 1995). First, absence declarations vary
according to the company and the country, depending on the methods
used to verify and/or compensate them. In some collective agreements,
absences for childcare are specifically available, whereas others require
parents to use their own sick days. Some require a medical certificate

right away, others later. Some employers put pressure on employees to come to work while sick, others do not.

Denominators for absence reports are also a source of confusion. Many reports contain no estimate at all for the number of hours normally worked by the employee, while others do not distinguish between full-time and part-time employees. Few reports specify how maternity leave has been treated, whether it is included in the numerator or the denominator (Deguire and Messing, 1995). Nevertheless, with all these problems, sickness absence, especially with a medical certificate, may prove a valuable indicator of problems in some jobs where accurate records are available or can be generated.

Other indicators which may be useful are those using indicators of sub-clinical pathological states such as pain symptoms, stress or biological alterations. These are states that normally do not impel the employee to leave her job, but that may be early indicators of health problems. Researchers have, for example, found sub-clinical neuropathy among microelectronics workers exposed to organic solvents (Mergler et al., 1991). Responses to medical interviews about menstrual irregularity can reveal early responses to variable work schedules (Messing et al., 1992). And various questionnaires have been developed in order to demonstrate stress responses among workers (Ilfeld, 1976).

The choice of indicators which will best reveal the hazards of women's jobs will depend on the characteristics of each jurisdiction. For example, a good indicator for Quebec may be a statistic which is not available in many other provinces or countries: the percentage of pregnancies where the worker has been granted preventive reassignment. In Quebec, the health and safety law allows a woman whose working conditions pose a danger for her foetus to request reassignment to a job without such dangers. (If reassignment is not possible, the worker is sent home at the equivalent of full pay.) Reassignment requires a medical and governmental determination that the job is dangerous. It can be seen from Table 7.2 that the lowest priority sectors are among those that are most dangerous for pregnant women, and that this method yields very different priorities even from those determined by women's rates of industrial accidents and diseases. I think this is because judgements about accident and disease recognition are coloured by sexism (Lippel, in press), which should not affect determinations of relative risk for pregnancy. Since very few risky working conditions affect only pregnant women, the rate of preventive reassignments may be a good way to determine priorities for prevention for all workers, by including hazards present in women's jobs.

Table 7.2   Reassignment of pregnant workers by priority sector,
Quebec, 1991

Sector, overall priority rank	Rank by accident rate, women 1991	Rank by industrial disease rate, women 1991	Rank by precautionary leave, 1991
1 Construction chemicals	6	6	6
2 Metallurgy, forestry manufacturing	1	1	2
3 Public administration, transportation, food processing	4	2	4
4 Commerce, textiles	3	3	1
5 Personal and commercial services, communications, printing	5	5	3
6 Medical and social services, teaching, insurance	2	4	2

The figures for the numerators are found in the *Annual Report* of the Quebec Occupational Health and Safety Commission, 1991. The denominators used came from *Statistics Canada* 1991, Table 1.

Research practices

Some research methods may lead researchers to underestimate risks in jobs held by women. One example is the widespread practice of 'adjusting for sex' in epidemiological studies (Mergler, 1995). Women have, for example, about 1.5–2 times the likelihood of reporting symptoms of 'sick building syndrome (SBS),' a set of respiratory, mucous membrane and central nervous system symptoms related to indoor air pollution. Most researchers deal with an excess of disease among women workers by using a mathematical procedure to 'correct' the percentages of illness among men to bring them up to women's levels (Franck *et al.*, 1993; Stenberg *et al.*, 1995). Others report that 'female sex' is a determinant of SBS without seeking to explain this finding (Skov *et al.*, 1989; Nelson *et al.*, 1995).

The reader is left with the interpretation that women are more likely to suffer SBS because of some psychological or physical weakness. Some scientists have not hesitated before leaping to the conclusion that women have more SBS because they more readily imagine things:

> Several epidemiologic features that might be used to help differentiate between building-associated illness caused by chemical exposure and that with a psychogenic origin... (4) characteristic personality profiles and age/sex distribution among patients. (Salvaggio, 1994, p. 369)

The impression is given that, when SBS affects a female workforce, scientists need not bother looking too long for chemical exposures.

Some scientists, however, have gone beyond this type of interpretation. Stenberg and Wall (1995) found that women office workers were more exposed to some of the known risk factors for SBS. They had less space allotted to them on average, which could affect both the efficiency of ventilation and the likelihood that they would be exposed to second-hand tobacco smoke in shared quarters. They were also more exposed to electrostatic effects from handling paper, photocopying and working at VDT screens for longer hours. It is possible, and even likely, that women may have specific diseases for biological reasons. There is some evidence that women may be more susceptible to multiple chemical sensitivities, a cause of SBS (Kipen et al., 1995). This should be investigated, but before concluding that special characteristics of women are responsible for differential rates of disease, alternative explanations must be eliminated.

The standard methods that have been used to adjust for sex in occupational health research have in fact concealed some risky working conditions. In 1987–88, a medical examination and questionnaire were administered to 558 men and 790 women as part of a study of seventeen poultry slaughterhouses and six canning factories. Women's and men's working conditions were very different and their sickness absences for musculoskeletal and respiratory illnesses were related to some of their specific working conditions: cold exposure, ill-adapted workstations and problems with their supervisors and co-workers. If men and women workers were combined into a single analysis while adjusting for sex, many of the associations operant for a single sex could no longer be seen (Messing et al., 1998).

Indicators for the hazards in women's work

Earlier in this chapter we suggested some possible indicators that could be used to make visible some occupational health effects of work in jobs usually held by women. We also need ways of characterising the jobs women do, indicators of the difficulties and risks involved. These tools are particularly necessary when jobs look easy or when they are characterised as 'light work' (Vézina *et al.*, 1992; Messing *et al.*, 1996). I will briefly present some indicators we have used in our studies of the work of factory and service workers. These were developed in consultation with the workers involved and were chosen to represent what they considered to be critical aspects of their jobs. Most of our indicators arise from observations of the work activity in situ. Observation is particularly necessary since many women workers underestimate the effort they exert. Union representatives tell us that women have lost their claims for compensation for repetitive strain injuries because they said 'I really don't do anything much' when asked to describe their jobs. Observations have enabled us to put a name to stressful aspects of women's jobs.

We have developed these indicators (and others not mentioned here) in the context of certain jobs in Quebec. Discussions with workers in other countries and other professions will surely produce other interesting indicators.

Physical aspects of work

For certain factory and service jobs it is important to consider repetitive gestures and to count the number of times a gesture is made, since repetitive movements can cause musculoskeletal disease. In a commercial bakery, women wrapped 7920 cakes per hour, with consequent strain on their upper limbs (Dumais *et al.*, 1993). Researchers have also counted repetitions by poultry processors (Vézina *et al.*, 1995) and others have counted characters per hour typed by data entry clerks (Billette and Piché, 1987).

Some repetitive gestures involve the use of force, and the total amount of force exerted may be an important determinant of joint inflammations. Vézina and colleagues used this indicator to compare the total force exerted by sewing machine operators to that, much smaller, exerted by men hired to move rolls of plastic in a factory (Vézina and Courville, 1992). Ergonomic standards for the workplace generally concern the types of lifting usually done by men, discrete heavy loads lifted all at once. A weight of 10kg should not be lifted more often than the limit set for the position in which the movement must be carried out. This standard setting is natural, because it is relatively easy to measure and control this type of lifting. It is not appropriate for those jobs, usually held by women, where small forces are exerted repeatedly, even though the cumulative force may be greater. For the type of lifting more common among women, limits should be put on the total force exerted in a day.

Light work/heavy work comparisons have been made in cleaning jobs and show that women in light work are exposed to postural constraints. For example, the sequence of objects dusted by women cleaners in a hospital (with the heights of the objects) was: table (81cm), television (196cm), table, telephone (81cm), lamp (to 188cm), table foot (11cm), chairs (46cm), window ledge (89cm), wall sphygmo-manometer (154cm) chair legs (to 46cm), oxygen apparatus (137cm). This sequence imposes rapid postural changes on the cleaners, who spent 74 per cent of their working time with the trunk flexed (Messing et al., 1996). Ergonomic standards do not cover the proportion of time spent in a flexed position, although such limits could be set.

Bank tellers, supermarket clerks and saleswomen are among the most common jobs for women in North America. Few of these workers are able to sit down while working. Seifert et al. (1997) observed bank tellers during 79 ten-minute intervals over three days and found that they spent 72 per cent of their time standing, with 73 per cent experiencing leg pain at least once a week. Again, ergonomic standards set no limit for the time spent standing, although such limits could be devised.

Cumulative load

School teachers in Quebec (and elsewhere) have very high levels of stress and burnout (Carpentier-Roy, 1991; Blais and Lachance, 1992; Gervais, 1993, p. 25). When we met with primary school teachers to discuss the reasons they felt exhausted and discouraged, they were unable to specify single factors for us to investigate. Instead, they referred to their 'global' workload. We were obliged to find a number of indicators which would reflect diverse aspects of their jobs (Messing et al., 1997). These included several indicators of environmental problems such as noise from the street or other classes, uncomfortable temperatures and too-low humidity levels, all of which distracted the pupils and made the teachers' jobs harder. We also counted the hours of work outside the paid work day and the numbers of procedures needed to arrange special help for children with emotional or learning problems. We counted the number of interruptions the teachers had to put up with and the number of simultaneous activities they had to engage in. Their emotional workload was rendered more difficult by public criticism of teachers, so we also compiled the tendencies of newspaper articles over a one-year period. When we examined working postures, we became aware that the teachers' physical workload was quite heavy. We therefore noted the percentage of time teachers flexed at the waist (more when children were younger and teachers bent over smaller desks) as well as time spent on their feet (almost all the time during class).

At first, union health and safety officers were sceptical: 'How can I ask inspectors who are accustomed to steel mills to worry about temperatures of 30 degrees Celsius, they'll laugh at me?' But most were eventually convinced that the long list of low-level stressors could, in combination, be responsible for the effects they were seeing on the workers' health. This example points up the necessity to consider multiple risk factors in context. Since most jobs held by women do not involve single, dramatic aggressors, more diffuse effects should be examined.

Balancing work and family

Health and safety legislation and practice usually recognise the standards necessary so that the worker can survive and keep working. Employers are required to provide rest breaks, water fountains, toilets and lunchtimes. But because regulations have evolved in relation to a male-pattern lifestyle, the need to meet family responsibilities has not always been included in labour standards. Workers, usually women, who must arrange childcare in order to work, bear this burden on their own. In order to make this workload visible, we compiled childcare arrangements made by telephone operators who received their schedules every Thursday for the week starting three days later, on the following Sunday (Prévost and Messing, 1997; Messing, 1998). Their starting and finishing times could change every day, and often did, so they had to make and remake their arrangements for childcare. Thirty operators with children under twelve kept records for two weeks. They made a total of 156 attempts to change their work hours (5.1 per operator) to meet family responsibilities. On the average, less than one of these succeeded. One operator made eighteen attempts without success.

The operators were relatively senior and had made regular arrangements for babysitters. But they had constantly to rearrange babysitting when they received their new hours. They made 212 rearrangements during the two weeks (4 per operator per work week). These results impelled the workers and their supervisors to develop ways to change the procedures used to set the schedules. We hope to have helped produce a permanent dialogue which could produce easier working conditions.

Conclusions

There are several reasons for the slow start in gathering information about the occupational health of women. A major reason is a question of academic disciplines. Medical and psychological specialists study health problems, while sociologists study women and work. Thus, clinicians are not aware of the data showing that women's and men's jobs are very different and may have different risks, while the social scientists are not always conscious of the health effects of the conditions they report.

Another important reason is that opportunities have been lacking for communication between scientists and workers. Scientists have thus been deprived of an important source of information on women's work and on their health problems. We have been particularly fortunate in being able to develop indicators through dialogue with women workers, in the context of an agreement between the Université du Québec and the three major Quebec trade unions (Messing and Mergler, 1993). Our projects are initiated through discussions with worker representatives and planned and carried out with their active collaboration. Results are discussed and validated with them. We recommend this procedure as a good way to develop scientific methods which can describe the effects of *work assigned* to women. An added benefit of contact with workers comes from the fact that when they describe their problems, they do not limit them by discipline, so cross-disciplinary collaboration becomes imperative. With the help of interdisciplinary and interclass collaboration, we feel sure that the health hazards in women's work can be rendered visible and, eventually, prevented.

Acknowledgements

We thank the workers involved in the studies for their collaboration and input and the Social Science and Humanities Research Council of Quebec for research support. Many of these studies were done in the framework of a partnership between the Université du Québec à Montréal and the women's committees of three Quebec labour unions (the Centrale de l'Enseignement du Québec, the Confédération des

Syndicats Nationaux and the Fédération des Travailleurs et Travailleuses du Québec), supported by the Conseil Québécois de la Recherche Sociale.

References

Alexanderson, K. (1998) 'Indicators for working women' in A. Kilborn, K. Messing and C. Thorbjornsson (eds) *Women's Health at Work*. Sweden: National Institute for Working Life.

Armstrong, P. and Armstrong, H. (1993) *The Double Ghetto*. 3rd edn. Toronto: McClelland & Stewart.

Billette, A. and Piché, J. (1987) 'Health problems of data entry clerks and related job stressors', *Journal of Occupational Medicine*, **29**: 942–8.

Blais, M. and Lachance, L. (1992). *Recherche-action sur la motivation et la qualité de vie au travail à la Commission scolaire de St-Jérôme*. Montréal, Québec: Université du Québec à Montréal.

Bourbonnais, R., Vinet, A., Vézina, M. and Gingras, S. (1992) 'Certified sick leave as a non-specific morbidity indicator: a case-referent study among nurses', *British Journal of Industrial Medicine*, **49**: 673–8.

Brooke, P.P. and Price, J.L. (1989) 'The determinants of employee absenteeism: an empirical test of a causal model', *Journal of Occupational Psychology*, **62**: 1–19.

Carpentier-Roy, M.C. (1991) *Organisation du travail et santé mentale chez les enseignantes et les enseignants du primaire et du secondaire*. Quebec: CEQ.

Chevalier, A., Luce, D., Blanc, C. and Goldberg, M. (1987) 'Sickness absence at the French National Electric and Gas Company', *British Journal of Industrial Medicine*, **44**: 101–10.

Commission de la Santé et de la Sécurité du Travail du Québec (CSST) (1993) *Rapport Annuel. Annexe Statistique*. Quebec: CSST.

Deguire, S. and Messing, K. (1995) 'L'étude de l'absence au travail a-t-elle un sexe?', *Recherches féministes*, **8**(2): 9–30.

Doyal, L. (1995) *What Makes Women Sick: Gender and the Political Economy of Health*. London: Macmillan.

Dumais, L., Messing, K., Seifert, A.M., Courville, J. and Vézina, N. (1993) 'Make me a cake as fast as you can: determinants of inertia and change in the sexual division of labour of an industrial bakery', *Work, Employment and Society*, **7**(3): 363–82.

Filkins, K. and Kerr, M.J. (1993) 'Occupational reproductive health risks', *Occupational Medicine: State of the Art Reviews*, **8**(4): 733–54.

Franck, C., Bach, E. and Skov, P. (1993) 'Prevalence of objective eye manifestations in people working in office buildings with different prevalences of the sick building syndrome compared with the general population', *International Archives of Occupational Environmental Health*, **65**: 65–9.

Gervais, M. (1993) *Bilan de santé des travailleurs québécois*. Montréal: Institut de recherche en santé et en sécurité du travail.

Goldberg, M. and Labrèche, F. (1996) 'Occupational risk factors for female breast cancer: a review', *Occupational and Environmental Medicine*, **53**: 145–56.

Guo, H., Tanaka, S., Cameron, L.L., Seligman, P.J., Behrens, V.J. Ger J., Wild, D.K. and Putz-Anderson, V. (1995) 'Back pain among workers in the United States: national estimates and workers at high risk', *American Journal of Industrial Medicine*, **28**: 591–602.

Ilfeld, F.W. (1976) 'Methodological issues in relating psychiatric symptoms to social stressors', *Psychological Reports*, **39**: 1251–8.

Kipen, H.M., Hallman, W., McNeil, K., Fiedler, Kathie and Fiedler, Nancy (1995) 'Measuring chemical sensitivity prevalence: a questionnaire for population studies', *American Journal of Public Health*, **85**(4): 574–7.

Laurin, G. (1991) *Féminisation de la main d'oeuvre: Impact sur la santé et la sécurité du travail*. Montréal, Québec: Commission de la Santé et de la Sécurité du Québec.

Lippel, K. (in press) 'Workers' compensation and stress: gender and access to compensation, *International Journal of Law and Psychiatry*.

Mergler, D. (1995) 'Adjusting for gender differences in occupational health studies' in K. Messing, B. Neis and L. Dumais (eds) *Invisible: Issues in Women's Occupational Health and Safety*. Charlottetown, PEI: Gynergy Books.

Mergler, D., Frenette, B., Legault-Béanger, S., Huel, G. and Bowler, R. (1991) 'Relationship between subjective symptoms of visual dysfunction and measurements of vision in a population of former microelectronics workers', *Journal of Occup. Med.* (Singapore), **3**(2): 75–83.

Messing, K. (1994) Women's occupational health and androcentric science. *Canadian Woman Studies*, **14**(3): 11–16.

Messing, K. (1998) *One-eyed Science: Occupational Health and Working Women*. Philadelphia: Temple University Press.

Messing, K. and Boutin, S. (1997) 'La reconnaissance des conditions difficiles dans les emplois des femmes et les instances gouvernementales en santé et en sécurité du travail', *Relations Industrielles/Industrial Relations*, **52** (2): 333–62.

Messing, K. and Mergler, D. (1993) 'Union and women's occupational health in Quebec' in L. Briskin and P. McDermott (eds), *Women Challenging Unions*. Toronto: University of Toronto Press.

Messing, K., Chatigny, C. and Courville, J. (1996) 'L'invisibilité du travail et la division léger/lourd dans l'entretien sanitaire: impact sur la santé et la sécurité du travail', *Objectif Prévention*, April–May 1996.

Messing, K., Seifert, A.M. and Escalona, E. (1997) 'The 120-second minute: using analysis of work activity to prevent psychological distress among elementary school teachers', *Journal of Occupational Health Psychology*, **2**(1): 45–62.

Messing, K., Neis, B. and Dumais, L. (eds) (1995) *Invisible: Issues in Women's Occupational Health and Safety*. Charlottetown, PEI: Gynergy Books.

Messing, K., Saurel-Cubizolles, M.-J., Kaminski, M. and Bourgine, M. (1992) 'Menstrual cycle characteristics and working conditions in poultry slaughterhouses and canneries', *Scand. J. Work Environ. Health*, **18**: 302–9.

Messing, K., Courville, J., Boucher, M., Dumais, L. and Seifert, A.M. (1994) 'Can safety risks of blue-collar jobs be compared by gender?', *Safety Science*, **18**: 95–112.

Messing, K., Tissot, F., Saurel-Cubizolles, M.-J., Kaminski, M. and Bourgine, M. (1998) 'Sex as a variable can be a surrogate for some working conditions:

factors associated with sickness absence'. *Journal of Occupational and Environmental Medicine*, **40**: 250–60.

Ministère de la santé et des services sociaux du Québec (1992) *La Politique de la santé et du bien-être*. Quebec: MSSS.

Nelson, N., Kaufman, J.D., Burt, J. and Karr, C. (1995) 'Health symptoms and the work environment in four nonproblem United States office buildings', *Scand. J. Work Environ. Health*, **21**: 51–9.

Prévost, J. and Messing, K. (1997) 'Quel horaire? What schedule? L'horaire de travail irrégulier des téléphonistes' in A. Soares (ed.), *Stratégies de résistances et travail des femmes*. Harmattan.: Montréal/Paris.

Pukkala, E., Auvinen, A. and Wahlberg, G. (1995) 'Incidence of cancer among Finnish airline cabin attendants, 1967–92', *British Medical Journal*, **311**: 649–52.

Robinson, J. C. (1989) 'Trends in racial equality and inequality and exposure to work-related hazards, 1968–1986', *AAOHN Journal*, **37**: 56–63.

Salvaggio, J. E. (1994) 'Psychological aspects of "environmental illness," "multiple chemical sensitivity", and building-related illness', *J. Allergy Clin. Immunol.*, **94**: 366–70.

Seifert, A.M., Messing, K. and Dumais, L. (1997) 'Star wars and strategic defense initiatives: work activity and health symptoms of unionized bank tellers during work reorganization', *International Journal of Health Services*, **27**(3): 455–77.

Skov, P., Valbjorn, O. and Pederson, B.V. (1989) 'The Danish indoor climate study group; influence of personal characteristics, job-related factors and psychosocial factors on the sick building syndrome', *Scand. J. Work Environ. Health*, **15**: 286–95.

Statistics Canada (1991) *Canada Census 1991. Catalogue 93–326, The Nation*. Ottawa: Statistics Canada.

Stellman, J. (1978) *Women's Work, Women's Health*. New York: Pantheon Books.

Stenberg, B., Eriksson, N., Mild, Kjell H.L., Höög, *et al.* (1995) 'Facial skin symptoms in visual display terminal workers. A case-referent study of personal, psychosocial, building- and VDT-related risk indicators', *International Journal of Epidemiology*, **24**(4): 796–803.

Stenberg, Berndt and Wall, Stig (1995) 'Why do women report "sick building symptoms" more often than men?' *Social Sciences and Medicine*, **40** (4): 491–5.

Vézina, N. and Courville, J. (1992) 'Integration of women into traditional masculine jobs', *Women and Health*, **18**(3) 97–118.

Vézina, N., Courville, J. and Geoffrion, L. (1995) 'Problèmes musculosquelettiques, caractéristiques des postes de travailleurs et des postes de travailleuses sur une chaîne de découpe de dinde' in K. Messing, B. Neis and L. Dumais (eds), *Invisible: Issues in Women's Occupational Health*. Charlottetown, Prince Edward Island: Gynergy Press.

Vézina, N., Tierney, D. and Messing, K. (1992) 'When is light work heavy? Components of the physical workload of sewing machine operators which may lead to health problems', *Applied Ergonomics*, **23**: 268–76.

Zahm, S.H., Pottern, L.M., Lewis, D.R., Ward, M.H. and White, D.W. (1994) 'Inclusion of women and minorities in occupational cancer epidemiological research', *Journal of Occupational Medicine*, **36**: 842–7.

8 IN THE HAND OR IN THE HEAD? CONTEXTUALISING THE DEBATE ABOUT REPETITIVE STRAIN INJURY (RSI)

Joyce E. Canaan

Several of the contributors to this volume have examined changing patterns of occupational risk linked with changing forms of work and employment in the global economy. This theme is explored in more detail in this chapter, which maps the rising incidence of a particular group of conditions collectively known as repetitive strain injury (RSI). The author demonstrates the importance of linking materialist and social constructionist accounts of occupational disease and injury. On the one hand, the growth of RSI can be linked to social and economic trends such as changes in work organisation and control of the labour process. On the other, the lack of medical and scientific consensus about the nature of RSI reveals the limitations of conventional reductionist models of disease that differentiate between 'real' illness residing in the body and 'unreal' illnesses originating in the mind. Neither of these approaches addresses the complexity of conditions such as RSI. Further, as in the case of a growing number of health problems, the insistence upon a dualist interpretation often serves to discredit and disempower the victims. This chapter presents a cogent case for a new understanding that recognises the links between mind and body in the causation of work-related ill health.

Introduction

Conventional understanding of repetitive strain injury (RSI) is strongly influenced by the belief that the cause of such conditions lies either in the body or in the mind but not in both. Meekosha and Jakubowicz (1991) suggest that this mind/body dualism overlooks:

> the interaction between occupational demands, psychological well being and physical symptoms. (1991, p. 35)

In order to prevent RSI, health and safety policies should therefore examine:

> not just the techniques of work, but also the hierarchies and structures which create dangerous stresses. (1991, p. 35)

The polarisation of the RSI debate is reflected in media reporting, illustrated for example by the title of an article which appeared in a leading British newspaper, 'In the Hand or Worker Hysteria' (Halliley, 1989).[1] The debate began in Australia in the 1980s, where RSI was initially recognised as a work-related injury and widely publicised as such. However, after a growing number of workers received compensation packages, a key legal case in 1987 'resolved' the debate by 'proving' that RSI was a psychological, rather than a physical, problem (Bammer and Martin, 1988, 1992; Reid and Reynolds, 1990; Meekosha and Jakubowicz, 1991).

This debate is about more than concepts. For if RSI is in the worker's body, then, it is argued – usually by employees, trade unionists and some doctors – that RSI is caused by work, and the employer should be liable for compensation payments. If no bodily evidence can be found, then – as other doctors, employers, insurers and the state have argued – RSI is due to individual psychological problems. This discredits the worker and effectively exempts the employer from accountability in relation to poor working conditions and compensation payments. Hence the definition of RSI, like that of other injuries and illnesses, has been shaped by powerful and sometimes diametrically opposed social, economic and political interests (Wright and Treacher, 1982; Lock and Gordon, 1988; Meekosha and Jakubowicz, 1991; Rosenberg and Golden, 1992).

While the Australian resolution of the RSI debate came down on the side of those who claimed that RSI was due to psychological causes, such a resolution has not (yet) occurred everywhere. Those of us committed to protecting workers' health and safety can therefore enter the debate about RSI so that different resolutions can be reached. However, we need not take the opposite view to that which was legally 'decided' in Australia – that is, we need not argue that RSI is solely a bodily based injury caused by work. For this ignores how mind and body can both be affected by work and may be simultaneously implicated in injuries such as RSI (Reid and Reynolds, 1990; Meekosha and Jakubowicz, 1991; Bammer and Martin, 1992).

The first section of this chapter highlights research that demonstrates the rising incidence of RSI, focusing mainly upon experiences within northern nations. This is not to suggest that RSI is confined to these nations, but rather is a consequence of the fact that in industrial countries there is greater reporting of occupational injury. Further, in these countries dramatic changes in working conditions and practices can be identified as underlining rising incidence rates. These changes in employment within industrialised societies are discussed in the second section. However, more research is needed to understand patterns of work and injury in southern countries which are increasingly affected by some of these global trends. The third section criticises the biomedical assumptions used by those on both sides of the RSI debate and suggests that alternative models are needed which address the social and political origins of work injury and which transcends the mind/body dualism that limits current understanding.

The rising incidence of RSI

RSI is an umbrella term for a number of conditions, only some of which are clinically recognised. These discrete manifestations include tenosynovitis (inflammation of the sheath surrounding a tendon), carpal tunnel syndrome (pain in the median nerve going from the forearm to the hand) and epicondylitis (inflammation of the area joining bone and muscle). However, it is estimated that up to 90 per cent of RSI sufferers experience other, more diffuse forms of RSI which are seldom recognised by official agencies and by the medical system (Labour Research Department, 1992; USDAW, 1992).

RSI symptoms include numbness, pain, pins and needles, muscle weakness, tenderness and loss or limit to movement. As many researchers have noted (Ireland, 1986; Brooks, 1987; Hopkins, 1989; Barton et al., 1992; Pheasant, 1992, 1993), the term RSI is in fact problematic, as the condition may not be caused by repetitive movement, may not fit medical definitions of strain and may not offer visible evidence of injury. Like Pheasant (1992), I use the term RSI because it is used by the media and the public, despite suggestions by official and trade union health and safety organisations that alternative terms, such as 'work-related upper limb disorders' or WRULD[2] be used. RSI has been described as:

> the single commonest cause of occupation-related time off work in the developed world. (Jefferies, 1992a, p. 41)

The World Health Organisation found that incidence of RSI doubled from 1988 to 1993 (Palmer, 1997). There is growing concern about RSI in Europe among those involved in workplace health and safety. In France, for example, RSI has increased significantly faster than other work-related injuries, from 212 reported cases in 1975 to 1040 in 1990 (Euro Review, 1994). Concommitantly, there was a 400 per cent increase in reported RSI among Finnish workers in the 1980s (Riihimaki, 1994).

Rising incidence rates have at times been checked by changes in work organisation. As early as the mid-1950s, Japanese workers newly using keyboards began getting RSI and by 1964 the Japanese Ministry of Labour issued guidelines restricting the number of hours and keystrokes that keypunchers performed (Maeda *et al.*, 1982; Miyake *et al.*, 1982; Nakaseko *et al.*, 1982; Ohara *et al.*, 1982; Silverstein, 1994). Similarly, as keyboards were introduced into Australia, those using these machines began to complain of RSI. Such complaints appeared to decline as ergonomic principles were applied to the relevant workplaces (Hopkins, 1989; Meekosha and Jakubowicz, 1991).[3]

These early lessons from Japan and Australia have not been generally applied elsewhere. In the USA, as early as 1983, the National Institute for Occupational Safety and Health (NIOSH) considered work-related musculoskeletal injuries generally as one of the top five categories of occupational injury. Yet the number of US workers reporting RSI continued to increase, rising fourfold from 1985 to 1989 (Stix, 1991). These disorders now account for 61 per cent of all new work-related illnesses in the USA (Silverstein, 1994, p. 36).

Similarly, in Britain the reported incidence of RSI has risen dramatically. A Department of Employment workplace survey in 1990 found that musculoskeletal problems accounted for about 550,000 lost working days, a doubling of the figure from 1983 (in Khilji and Smithson, 1994, p. 95). Consequently, employer's liability costs rose during this period, trebling between 1984 and 1988 (Jefferies, 1992b, p. 43). These claims were seen as likely 'to continue unless preventative action is taken now' (Jefferies, 1992b, p. 43). Such action has not been taken: by 1995 a still growing number of RSI claims led to an increase in employers' liability insurance costs (*Occupational Health,* April 1995, p. 116).

Reorganising production

The rising incidence of RSI among northern workers can be linked to changes in the organisation and management of paid employment. During the twentieth century, the introduction of systems known as Fordism and Taylorism have profoundly intensified the physical and psychosocial[4] pressures of work (Braverman, 1974). More recently, additional transformations have led to considerable job losses and have heightened workers' anxiety and insecurity. These processes, which initially impacted on blue-collar workers, have increasingly affected white-collar workers too.

Fordism refers to the new way of life experienced by many workers during the early twentieth century after Henry Ford introduced a number of innovations into US production. These included the assembly line, which rationalised and mechanised production, and the standardisation of parts assembled along this line. Fordism was said to enable economies of scale, dramatically increasing the number of goods produced. While such factories required great capital outlay on machinery, employers recouped their expenses and made massive profits by producing and selling large volumes of goods (Allen, 1992; Webster and Robins, 1993; Amin, 1994; Kumar, 1995).

These changes were accompanied by the introduction of Taylorist scientific management principles. These were used to ensure that the large numbers of goods produced were made by using workers' bodies as fully and efficiently as possible. This usage required increased managerial control over workers. Managers gained this control by acting 'as information specialists – ideally as monopolists – as close observers, analysts and planners of the production process' (Webster and Robins, 1993, p. 245).

By the second decade of the postwar era, Fordism and Taylorism together increasingly deskilled many manual workers, who were performing smaller and more repetitive tasks. These tasks extracted more labour from employees who were more closely monitored by the growing layers of management. Employees initially ignored this monitoring because employers, needing labourers and consumers, recognised that paying workers well would encourage greater productivity and consumption (Sewell and Wilkinson, 1992; Elam, 1994).

However, by the late 1960s employers found Fordism and Taylorism problematic for several reasons.

First, both processes required a flowline of continuous, efficient production, but in practice this flowline was neither continuous nor efficient. This was partly due to workers seeking to control their cycle time – the time designated to complete a task – by doing it more quickly than was demanded in order to gain some time for themselves as well as some control over their increasingly deskilled and monitored work. In addition, their growing confidence, due to their mass numbers in factories and their improved pay and outside conditions, helped them recognise that they had made a Faustian bargain with management in the early postwar era by agreeing to 'higher wages in return for [greater] management control of production' (Murray in Allen, 1992, p. 215). They left jobs they disliked (since labour was relatively scarce and other jobs were available), and resisted or struck against management strategies they opposed. Their dissent slowed the flowline, hindering capital's ability to maximise profits from production and consumption (Allen, 1992; Sewell and Wilkinson, 1992; Aronowitz and DiFazio, 1994; Tomaney, 1994).

Second, under Fordism and Taylorism the links between production and consumption, and supply and demand were inefficient. When demand was lower than supply, goods were stored rather than sold, which added to capital's costs and disrupted the flowline from production to consumption. In addition, product defects were discovered *after* rather than *during* production, which wasted many workers' efforts, thereby adding more to capital's costs. Finally, as more northern nations used Fordist and Taylorist principles to develop factories, competition increased. This required companies to lower the price of their goods, which was difficult, given their high postwar wage agreements with unions.

From the mid-1970s the development of informational technologies offered employers new means of responding to these tensions. These techonologies enabled radical transformations, streamlining production and reducing the numbers of workers needed. Further, these transformations made it easier for capital to shift or expand factories between nations. Northern companies benefited from conditions in southern nations where governments, 'desperate not for development as such but to end the unemployment that threatens their regimes' (Sivanandan, 1990, p. 181), often agreed to quell worker dissatisfaction with their national security forces (Sivanandan, 1996).

The increased mobility of capital and the reduced need for labour also impacted on northern factory workers. They began to find that if they caused unrest, their employers might move production to a nation with a more 'docile' and cheap workforce (Sherman, 1995; Robinson, 1996; Wilkin, 1996). In addition, they found that some of their jobs were being eliminated. For example, 33 per cent of US workers had manual jobs in the 1950s, compared to less than 17 per cent by 1995 (Rifkin, 1995). For those who remained in employment, pay and conditions were being eroded as productivity was increasing (Silverstein, 1994; Dahrendorf, 1995; European Work Hazards Network, 1995; Dunkerley, 1996; Sivanandan, 1996).

New informational technologies have also been introduced into middle-class jobs since the early 1980s. These technologies have streamlined such jobs and made them more insecure and stressful in the same way that they have heightened job insecurity and stress in working-class jobs. For example, in the UK there is now thought to be a bottom tier of 30 per cent who are 'unemployed and economically inactive', a middle 30 per cent in 'newly insecure' jobs and 'the top 40 per cent [who] hold relatively secure jobs – whose security is being eroded as 1 per cent annually are squeezed out of this sector' (Hutton, 1995, pp. 2–3).

However, it is not new informational technologies alone that have eroded workers' pay, conditions and security. Rather, these processes began with new management strategies introduced in early postwar Japanese factories that spread to other northern nations from the early 1980s (Elam, 1994). In Japan, the state stopped high levels of trade union dissent by establishing company unions in which union members were carefully chosen from among those who agreed with management's aim of 'rationaliz[ing] production and intensify[ing] work processes' (Tomaney, 1994, p. 168). This dramatically increased productivity. The profits of Nissan for example, rose 55 fold in the twenty years after an independent union was replaced by one organised by the company (Yamamoto in Garrahan and Stewart, 1992, p. 10).

Japanese corporations also rationalised factory production by implementing just-in-time production (JIT) and total quality control (TQC). JIT aimed to produce just enough goods to meet market demand while TQC aimed to control production by producing goods without defects. By producing just enough high quality goods as were necessary, the flowline within production and between production and consumption could be continuously moving so that capital could appropriate workers' labour as fully as possible. The need to store unwanted goods was eliminated and supply shortages were overcome by having employees work longer, harder and faster when supply demands were high. Thus factory workers were utilised more intensively and production, delivery and consumption were better coordinated – enabling greater profits for owners and managers (Sewell and Wilkinson, 1992; Berggren, 1993; Tomaney, 1994).[5]

The impact of new production methods on workers' health

While JIT and TQC *seemed* to solve key problems of Fordist and Taylorist production (Womack *et al.*, 1990), a growing literature suggests that this solution benefits employers and managers at the expense of employees who face increased stress and health problems. When JIT was introduced at the Mazda car plant in Michigan in 1987, for example, workers were 'busy 57 seconds out of every minute, in contrast to 45 seconds at plants owned by the Big Three [US] automobile makers' (Stix, 1991, p. 83). Not surprisingly, Mazda workers had 'an unusually high incidence' of carpal tunnel syndrome (Berggren, 1993, p. 177) attributed to the production system 'which elicits maximum efficiency from workers and machinery' (Wokutch in Berggren, 1993, p. 178).

JIT and TQC also reportedly democratised the factory floor, as employees worked in teams, striving continuously to improve their productive roles. Teamwork was seen by some as giving workers more responsibility over their work and enabling them to respond to problems as they occurred rather than going through multiple layers of bureaucracy (Garrahan and Stewart, 1992; Berggren, 1993). These teamwork strategies have also allowed management to encourage workers to monitor their own and others' performance. At daily meetings team members discuss the previous day's productivity and consider how to improve completion times in the future. Management thus encourages workers to watch over themselves and each other using techniques that Parker and Slaughter dub 'management-by-stress' (in Garrahan and Stewart, 1992; Sewell and Wilkinson, 1992). This monitoring is bolstered by new informational surveillance systems that check work quality and specify the team, and sometimes the individual, responsible for problems (Garrahan and Stewart, 1992; Sewell and Wilkinson, 1992).

Studies suggest that this intensification of work considerably erodes workers' control over their working practices and thereby heightens the risk of injury. Workers performing the same minute movements with barely a rest between them have a high risk of getting RSI (Maeda *et al.*, 1982; Nakaseko *et al.*, 1982). A recent study of French female assembly workers found that these women were performing tasks which doubled in pace from 1984 to 1991 – at a time when the incidence of RSI was growing nationally (Kilbom, 1994). Swedish women assemblers in electronics, an area of work known to involve increasingly smaller and more repetitive activities, were found to be twenty times more likely than other workers to get RSI (Euro Review, 1994). These findings indicate that workers' minds and bodies are both affected by the intensification of work and the erosion of control over work processes.

Studies now also suggest that some white-collar workers' bodies are also being harnessed to machines in ways that use their labour more fully and, concomitantly, erode their control over their work. The introduction of computers into office work, for example, eliminates the need for keyboard workers to break for a carriage return at the end of a line and for a new sheet of paper at the end of a page. In addition, the lesser pressure of computer keys relative to typewriters enables keyboard workers to type more quickly, thereby repeating similar motions more frequently (Barrer, 1991; Pheasant, 1993). As keyboard work can be done so rapidly, some workers are requested to type at high keystroke rates with few breaks over long time periods. This ignores studies that have found that keyboard workers are more likely to get RSI as high work rates are set, breaks are lessened, and control over work decreases (Maeda *et al.*, 1982, Nakaseko *et al.*, 1982; Stone, 1984; Buckle, 1994).

While recent (1992) European legislation specified employers' health and safety responsibilities to their visual display unit (VDU) users, some employers have tried to avoid meeting these responsibilities (Palmer, 1997). Thus, a growing number of white-collar workers are now finding that, like manual labourers, their work pace is intensifying. In addition, as computers now have managerial monitoring incorporated into them by measuring the number of keystrokes produced per hour and the percentage of each hour worked, white-collar workers, too, are facing heightened productivity demands and heightened scrutiny – literally, at their fingertips – as their control over their labour lessens.

This analysis suggests that the increasing 'flexibility' of work improves efficiency of production for employers, but brings increased health and safety risks for workers. Both blue- and white-collar workers face heightened surveillance and decreased control as their job insecurity grows. These factors raise psychosocial stress at work more than before at the same time as the physical stresses are increasing. As Wall has noted, such stress 'may cause workers to tense their muscles unnecessarily and working with tensed arms or hands may in turn cause injury (in Hopkins, 1989, p. 257). Stress, a factor commonly thought to be singularly located in the mind, can therefore impact directly on the body, increasing the risk of RSI (Maeda *et al.*, 1982; Nakaseko *et al.*, 1982; Ohara *et al.*, 1982; Hagberg, 1994; Buckle and Hoffman, 1996).

Biomedical debates about RSI

In responding to the rising incidence of RSI, it is imperative that medical workers recognise both the physical and the psychosocial stresses of work. Yet biomedicine, the dominant medical system of the north, presumes that work can legitimately impact on the body alone. This presumption serves to discredit many sufferers, particularly those with diffuse RSI symptoms. They are seen as suffering from psychological problems as opposed to 'real' occupational illness. The assumption that body and mind are distinct entities, with 'real' illness located in the body, allows biomedicine to limit how much of the self illness or injury can inhabit (Scheper-Hughes and Lock, 1987; Gordon, 1988).

A further assumption of biomedicine is that while patient symptoms may guide the diagnosis of illness, disease is only confirmed by the presence of clinically visible signs. Further, 'real' disease is only recognised when a specific disease entity or agent causing illness or injury is found in the patient's body. This is known as 'the doctrine of specific aetiology' (Rosenberg, 1992a; Nettleton, 1995; Cooper, 1997). If a clear cause can be found (for example, from an X-ray which shows a broken bone), then the illness or injury being diagnosed is legitimated.

Within the process of diagnosis, greater weight is given to the doctor's *observation* of visible signs than to the patients' *experience* of symptoms (Smith, 1981), which indicates that, as Scheper-Hughes and Lock note, '[t]he medical gaze is, then, a controlling gaze' (1987, p. 27). This controlling aspect of biomedicine has increasingly been challenged. Rather than diagnosing and treating illness in a detached, objective and universally applicable way, biomedicine and its key assumptions are seen to be shaped by 'hidden cultural scaffolding and social processes' (Gordon, 1988, p. 20; see also Wright and Treacher, 1982; Scheper-Hughes and Lock, 1987; Rosenberg and Golden, 1992).

The process of diagnosing an illness or injury is therefore more complex than the medical model suggests, involving struggles between competing interests and perspectives (Markowitz and Rosner, 1992; Rosenberg, 1992a; Nettleton, 1995; Cooper, 1997). For example, diagnosis of myalgic encephalomyelitis (ME) is made difficult by the absence of clinical signs, the lack of availability of diagnostic tests and the failure to identify a specific aetiology. Consequently, psychiatrists and people with ME have long debated whether ME is a 'real' illness, indicative of a problem with a person's body, or an 'unreal' illness, indicative instead of a problem with their mind.

This political debate between interest groups is heightened in the case of occupational illness or injury where the process of defining disease can legitimate or delegitimate not just symptoms and treatments but the beliefs and claims of workers and employers (Rosenberg, 1992b, p. 185). Liability for damaging working practices and compensation payments are in question and the stakes are literally higher in occupational than non-occupational illness or injury.

Despite these problems, occupational health policies continue to reflect the medical model. In Britain, for example, an employee only receives compensation for RSI if she or he can provide medical evidence that work alone has caused their symptoms (Robin Thompson and Partners, Brian Thompson and Partners, 1994). Compensation is therefore limited to the small number of sufferers whose symptoms are seen to be legitimised by clinical evidence.

As Australian social scientists (Bammer and Martin, 1988, 1992; Reid and Reynolds, 1990; Meekosha and Jakubowicz, 1991) have noted, there have been two sides to the RSI debate. Adherents to the 'standard medical view' (Bammer and Martin, 1988, 1992) consider RSI a 'real', bodily based injury that can be caused by work. Alternatively, critics of this view suggest that RSI can be explained, at least in part, by psychological factors.

Adherents of the standard view emphasise the importance of clinical signs of injury, and a variety of tests is thought to confirm patients' symptoms as RSI (Ferguson, 1971; Stone, 1984; Fry, 1986; Armstrong et al., 1987). Some adherents claim to have found evidence of pathology in discrete body parts (Armstrong et al., 1987; Herrick and Herrick, 1987; Dennett and Fry, 1988).

Holders of the standard medical view maintain that the cause of RSI lies in the workplace not the worker (Armstrong et al., 1987; Herrick and Herrick, 1987; Silverstein, 1994). However, their arguments are limited by a failure fully to explore how the workplace has changed in recent years. New technologies and working practices do not simply introduce additional stresses into the workplace as prior technologies have done (see, for example, Silverstein, 1994), but now enable the extraction of more labour from workers' bodies, fuller monitoring of this labour and, importantly, a greater erosion of workers' control over their jobs than before (Stone, 1984; Frankenhauser, 1994).

Critics of the standard medical view point out that the physiological model of RSI fails to account for experiences of the vast majority of sufferers, although they accept that 10 per cent of cases can be confirmed as clinical disease (Ireland, 1986; Wright, 1987; Miller and Topliss, 1988; Hadler, 1990). Rather than attempting to broaden the medical model, they focus instead on the psychological causes of diffuse RSI, suggesting that the problem lies within the worker's psyche. However, while they demand stringent clinical evidence to prove physical injury, they fail to provide equally stringent evidence to prove their assertion of psychological problems (Bammer and Martin, 1992). There are other inconsistencies in the position of these critics. For instance they maintain that in cases where RSI symptoms cannot be confirmed biomedically, psychological and social factors *together* may cause symptoms. Thus, while they – as well as holders of the standard medical view – look to a singular cause of discrete RSI, they look to multiple causes to explain diffuse RSI. Neither group explains why multiple factors can influence RSI if it is located in the mind but not if it is in the body.

The multiple factors cited as causing diffuse RSI include, importantly, patients' personalities. While some critics acknowledge that new technology, job insecurity and other sources of stress may contribute to RSI, others suggest that only some workers 'choose' to emphasise dissatisfaction in this way (Miller and Topliss, 1988; Hadler, 1990). Hence, workers are blamed and the impact of recent transformations in the workplace on workers' minds and bodies is ignored. Some critics further suggest that people with diffuse RSI heighten pain symptoms because of personal failings such as lack of confidence, anxiety and job dissatisfaction (Hadler, 1990, p. 40). Indeed, some critics maintain that RSI involves a 'hysterical conversion disorder' (Ireland, 1986, p. 415; see also Awerbuch, 1985; Lucire, 1986a, 1986b) where people with boring, repetitive and low paid jobs – who, coincidentally, are mostly women – convert psychosocial dissatisfaction into physical pain.

Such notions clearly fail to recognise the material basis for RSI. Evidence suggests, for example, that it is the fact that women are more likely than men to be assigned to small, repetitive jobs which increase their likelihood of getting RSI (Stone, 1984; Meekosha, 1986; Reid and Reynolds, 1990). Because women are also those who perform most housework, which involves small, repetitive movements before and/or after doing paid work, it is not surprising that the incidence of RSI is higher for women than men (see Meekosha, 1986; Segal, 1990).

Critics also claim that RSI is an iatrogenic illness, arguing that workers are encouraged by the medicalised term RSI to link normal aches and pains caused by work with serious injury (Brooks, 1987; Cleland, 1987; Wright, 1987; Miller and Topliss, 1988; Hadler, 1990).

The compensation system is seen as reinforcing this problem, encouraging people to believe, wrongly, that they have RSI and discouraging efforts at rehabilitation. These critics argue for an alternative term to RSI that avoids the suggestive link between work and injury. However, this would limit the extent to which people view accepted activities as harmful or physical sensations as indicative of underlying damage. In addition, there is a danger of implying that people with diffuse RSI are particularly suggestible and, at worst, simply motivated by financial gain.

These critics of the standard medical view fail to suggest a satisfactory alternative framework for explaining RSI. Rather than attributing RSI either to the mind or the body, we need to recognise that psychological and physical illness or injury can both stem from multiple factors. Attention needs to be paid to the ways in which newly intensified pressures on workers' minds and bodies increase their likelihood of injury. Yet the health implications of dramatic transformations in the workplace have received relatively little attention in the literature on RSI.

In developing a new understanding of occupational health problems, the importance of names and language in defining, explaining and legitimating or delegitimating illness or injury needs to be acknowledged. This suggests that, with regard to RSI in particular, we need a term which acknowledges that disease can be simultaneously caused by work and yet also be structured in complex ways in the minds and bodies of the workers involved.

Conclusion

This chapter has examined the biomedical debate about RSI in the context of research linking rising injury rates to recent changes in employment. An examination of these literatures suggests that those seeking to highlight the impact of the intensification of the struggle between workers and managers could do so more effectively if they considered the effects of work on health. The scale and damage caused by RSI suggests that these effects are profound.

The chapter has argued that biomedical accounts of RSI – and, indeed, of illness and injury more generally – are limited. For neither holders of the standard medical view of RSI nor their critics have seriously considered how recent changes in working conditions and practices are damaging our minds and bodies. Rather than arguing that RSI is either 'in the hand or in the head', we need to recognise that mind and body are interconnected and that work increasingly impacts on both of these parts of our selves.

Notes

1   Although I use the term 'RSI' in the singular, many conditions fall within this definition, as noted earlier.

2   Some commentators, for example the UK Health and Safety Commission, now speak of 'WRULDs' to acknowledge that occupational and non-occupational factors may both be present (*Occupational Health Review* August/September, 1990, p. 3. However, the term WRULDs ignores RSI in the lower limbs.

3   This 'decline' must in fact be read with caution. In New South Wales alone RSI is still the 'second largest industrial disease' (*OOS News*, March 1994, p. 1). In addition, government statistics on the incidence of RSI are no longer kept and compensation payments are more difficult to obtain (Willis, 1994).

4   I use the term 'psychosocial' rather that 'psychological' to emphasise that workers' social milieu impacts on them.

5   Some argue, however, that this increased competition is eliminating many companies (see Dunkerley, 1996; Garrahan and Stewart, 1992).

Acknowledgements

I would like to thank Paul Grant, the editors and Bob Whiskens for guiding my reading and for commenting on an earlier draft.

References

Allen, J. (1992) 'Post-industrialism and post-Fordism' in S. Hall, D. Held and T. McGree (eds), *Modernity and Its Futures*. Cambridge: Polity.

Amin, A. (ed.) (1994) *Post-Fordism: A Reader*. Oxford: Blackwell.

Armstrong, T.J., Fine, L.J., Goldstein, S.A., Lifshitz, Y.R. and Silverstein, B.A. (1987) 'Ergonomic considerations in hand and wrist tendinitis', *The Journal of Hand Surgery*, **12A**(5) Part 2, September: 830–7.

Aronowitz, S. and DiFazio, W. (1994) *The Jobless Future: Sci-Tech and the Dogma of Work*. London: University of Minnesota Press.

Awerbuch, M. (1985) '"RSI" or "Kangaroo Paw"', *Medical Journal of Australia*, **142**: 237–8.

Bammer, G. and Martin, B. (1988) 'The arguments about RSI: an examination', *Community Health Studies*, **12**(3): 348–80.

Bammer, G. and Martin B. (1992) 'Repetition strain injury in Australia: medical knowledge, social movement and de facto partisanship', *Social Problems*, **39**(3) August: 219–37.

Barrer, S.J. (1991) 'Gaining the upper hand on carpal tunnel syndrome', *Occupational Health and Safety*, January: 38–43.

Barton, N.J., Hooper, G., Noble, J. and Steel, W.M. (1992) 'Occupational causes of disorders in the upper limb', *British Medical Journal*, (304): 309–11.

Berggren, C. (1993) 'Lean production – the end of history?', *Work, Employment and Society*, **7**(2): 189–212.

Braverman, H. (1974) *Labour and Monopoly Capital: The Degradation of Work in the Twentieth Century*. New York: Monthly Review.

Brooks, P. (1987) 'Repetition strain injury', *The Lancet*, September 26: 738.

Brooks, P. (1993) 'Repetition strain injury does not exist as a separate medical condition', *British Medical Journal*, **307**(20 November): 1298.

Buckle, P. (1994) 'Work-related upper limb disorders and keyboard work: why we may lose the battle', *New Epidemics in Occupational Health*, People and Work Research Reports Vol. 1, Finnish Institute of Occupational Health, Helsinki.

Buckle, P. and Hoffman, J. (1996) 'Work-related upper limb disorders: a guide to assessing WRULDs', produced as part of the TUC WRULD Campaign. Guildford: Ergonomics Research Unit, University of Surrey.

Cleland, L.G. (1987) '"RSI": a model of social iatrogenesis', *Medical Journal of Australia*, **147** (7 September): 236–39.

Cooper, L. (1997) 'Professional closure and resistance in the ME controversy', unpublished paper given at the 1997 British Sociological Association conference, University of York, April.

Dahrendorf, R. (1995) 'Preserving prosperity', *New Statesman & Society*, **15/29** (December 1995): 36–7.

Dennett, X. and Fry, H.J.J. (1988) 'Overuse syndrome: a muscle biopsy study', *The Lancet*, **I** (April 23): 905–7.

Dunkerley, M. (1996) *The Jobless Economy?: Computer Technology in the World of Work*. Cambridge: Polity.

Elam, M. (1994) 'Puzzling out the post-Fordist debate: technology, markets and institutions', in A. Amin (ed.) *Post-Fordism: A Reader*. Oxford: Blackwell.

Euro Review (1994) *Repetitive Strain Injury*. Dublin: European Foundation for the Improvement of Living and Working Conditions.

European Work Hazards Network (1995) *Deregulation of Health and Safety Legislation in Europe. A Presentation to Members of the European Parliament*. Brussels: EWHN.

Ferguson, D. (1971) 'Repetition injuries in process workers', *Medical Journal of Australia*, (2): 408–12.

Frankenhauser, M. (1994) 'Psychosocial factors and occupational health' in J. Rantanen, S. Lentinen, R. Kalimo, H. Nordman, H. Vainio, and E. Viikari-Juntura (eds), *New Epidemics in Occupational Health*. People and Work Research Reports Vol. 1, Finnish Institute of Occupational Health, Helsinki.

Fry, H.J.H. (1986) 'Overuse syndrome in musicians: prevention and management', *The Lancet*, **II** (September 27): 728–31.

Garrahan, P. and Stewart, P. (1992) *The Nissan Enigma: Flexibility at Work in a Local Economy*. London: Mansell.

Gordon, D. (1988) 'Tenacious assumptions in western medicine' in M. Lock and D. Gordon (eds), *Biomedicine Examined*. London: Kluwer Academic.

Hagberg, M. (1994) 'Pathomechanisms of work-related musculoskeletal disorders' in J. Rantanen, S. Lentinen, R. Kalimo, H. Nordman, H. Vainio, and E. Viikari-Juntura (eds), *New Epidemics in Occupational Health*. People and

Work Research Reports Vol. 1, Finnish Institute of Occupational Health, Helsinki.

Hadler, N.M. (1990) 'Cumulative trauma disorders: an iatrogenic concept', *Journal of Occupational Medicine*, **32**(1) January: 38–41.

Halliley, M.(1989) 'In the hand or worker hysteria?', *The Independent* 29 August, 13.

Herrick, R.T. and Herrick, S.K. (1987) 'Thermography in the detection of carpel tunnel syndrome and other compressive neuropathies', *The Journal of Hand Surgery*, **12A**(5) Part 2, September: 943–49.

Hopkins, A. (1989) 'The social construction of repetition strain injury', *Australian and New Zealand Journal of Sociology*, **25**(2) August: 239–59.

Hutton, W. (1995) 'High risk strategy', *Guardian*, 30 October (Section 2): 2–3.

Ireland, D.C.R. (1986) 'Repetition strain injury', *Australian Family Physician*, **15**(4) April: 415–18.

Jefferies, H. (1992a) 'Hands-on workplace protection', *Safety Management*, September: 41.

Jefferies, H. (1992b) 'Dramatic rise in ULD insurance claims', *Safety Management*, September: 43.

Khilji, N. and Smithson, S. (1994) 'Repetitive strain injury in the UK: soft tissues and hard issues', *International Journal of Information Management*, April: 95–108.

Kilbom, A. (1994) 'Repetitive work of the upper extremity Part I: Guidelines for practitioners' in A. Kilbom and A. Mital (eds), *International Journal of Industrial Ergonomics*, **14**: 51–7.

Kumar, K. (1995) *From Post-Industrial to Post-Modern Society: New Theories of the Contemporary World*. Oxford: Blackwell.

Labour Research Department (1992) *RSI: A Trade Unionists' Guide*. London: Labour Research Department.

Lock, M. and Gordon, D. (eds) (1988) *Biomedicine Examined*. London: Kluwer Academic.

Lucire, Y. (1986a) 'Neurosis in the Workplace', *Medical Journal of Australia*, **145**: 323–27.

Lucire, Y. (1986b) 'RSI: when emotions are converted', *Safety Australia*, February (9): 8–12.

Maeda, K., Horiguchi, S. and Hosodawa, M. (1982) 'History of the studies of occupational cervicobrachial disorder in Japan and remaining problems', *Journal of Human Ergology*, **11**: 17–29.

Markowitz, G. and Rosner, D. (1992) 'The illusion of medical certainty: silicosis and the politics of industrial disability, 1930–1960' in C.E. Rosenberg and J. Golden (eds), *Framing Disease: Studies in Cultural History*. New Brunswick: Rutgers University Press.

Meekosha, H. (1986) 'Eggshell personalities strike back – a response to the bosses' doctors on RSI', *Refractory Girl*, **29** (May): 2–6.

Meekosha, H. and Jakubowicz, A. (1991) 'Repetitive strain injury: the rise and fall of an "Australian" disease', *Critical Social Policy*, **11** (Summer): 18–37.

Miller, M.H. and Topliss, D.J. (1988) 'Chronic upper limb syndrome (repetitive strain injury) in the Australian workplace: a systematic cross sectional rheumatological study of 229 patients', *Journal of Rheumatology*, **15**(11): 1705–12.

Miyake, S., Himeno, J. and Hosokawa, H. (1982) 'Clinical features of occupational cervicobrachial disorder (OCD)', *Journal of Human Ergology*, **11**: 109–17.

Nakaseko, M., Tokunaga, R. and Hosokawa, M. (1982) 'History of occupational cervicobrachial disorder in Japan', *Journal of Human Ergology*, **11**: 7–16.

Nettleton, S. (1995) *The Sociology of Health and Illness*. Cambridge: Polity.

Occupational Health Review (1990) 'Lessons of Australia's "RSI" epidemic', August/September: 2–5.

Occupational Health (1995) 'Concern over RSI claims', April, 116.

Occupational Overuse Syndrome News (1994) 'Justice for all?', March: 1.

Ohara, H., Itani, T. and Aoyama, H. (1982) 'Prevalence of occupational cervicobrachial disorder among different occupational groups in Japan', *Journal of Human Ergology*, **11**: 55–63.

Palmer, C. (1997) 'Office safety: are you aching for change?', *Observer Business Section*, 19 October: 9.

Pheasant, S. (1992) 'Does RSI exist?', *Occupational Medicine*, **42**: 167–8.

Pheasant, S. (1993) 'Reply' to A.J.M. Slovak, 'Does RSI exist?', *Occupational Medicine*, **43**: 53–4.

Reid, J. and Reynolds, L. (1990) 'Requiem for RSI: the explanation and control of an occupational epidemic', *Medical Anthropology Quarterly*, **4**(2) June: 162–90.

Rifkin, J. (1995) 'The end of work?', *New Statesman & Society*, 9 June: 18–25.

Riihimaki, H. (1994) 'Statistics of occupational diseases – a mirror of morbidity from repetitive strain injuries?' in J. Rantanen, S. Lentinen, R. Kalimo, H. Nordman, H. Vainio and E. Viikari-Juntura (eds), *New Epidemics in Occupational Health*. People and Work Research Reports Vol. 1, Finnish Institute of Occupational Health, Helsinki.

Robinson, I. (1988) *Multiple Sclerosis*. London: Routledge.

Rosenberg, C.E. (1992a) 'Framing disease: illness, society, and history' in C.E. Rosenberg and J. Golden (eds), *Framing Disease: Studies in Cultural History*. New Brunswick: Rutgers University Press.

Rosenberg, C.E. (1992b) 'Introduction' to G. Markowitz and D. Rosner, 'The illusion of medical certainty' in C.E. Rosenberg, and J. Golden (eds), *Framing Disease: Studies in Cultural History*, New Brunswick: Rutgers University Press.

Rosenberg, C.E. and Golden, J. (1992) (eds) *Framing Disease: Studies in Cultural History*. New Brunswick: Rutgers University Press.

Robinson, W.I. (1996) 'Globalization: Nine themes on our epoch', *Race and Class*, **38**(2): 13–52.

Scheper-Hughes, N. and Lock, M.M. (1987) 'The mindful body: a prolegomenon to future work in medical anthropology', *Medical Anthropology Quarterly*, **1**: 6–41.

Segal, L. (1990) *Slow Motion: Changing Masculinities, Changing Men*. London: Virago.

Sewell, G. and Wilkinson, B. (1992) '"Someone to watch over me": surveillance, discipline and the just-in-time labour process', *Sociology*, **20**(2): 271–89.

Sherman, B. (1995) 'The end of work as we know it?', *New Statesman*, 27 October: 27–31.

Silverstein, B.A. (1994) 'New work-related musculoskeletal epidemics: a review' in J. Rantanen, S. Lentinen, R. Kalimo, H. Nordman, H. Vainio and E. Viikari-Juntura (eds) *New Epidemics in Occupational Health*. People and Work Research Reports Vol. 1, Finnish Institute of Occupational Health, Helsinki.

Sivanandan, A. (1990) *Communities of Resistance: Writings on Black Struggles for Socialism*. London: Verso.

Sivanandan, A. (1996) 'Heresies and prophecies: the social and political fall-out of the technological revolution: an interview', *Race and Class*, **37**(4): 1–11.

Smith, B.E. (1981) 'Black lung: the social production of disease' in N. Navarro and D.M. Berman (eds), *Health and Work under Capitalism: An International Perspective*. Farmingdale, NY: Baywood.

Stix, G. (1991) 'Handful of pain', *Scientific American*, May: 82–3.

Stone, W.E. (1984) 'Occupational repetitive strain injuries', *Australian Family Physician*, **13**(9) September.

Thompson, Robin and Partners, and Thompson, Brian and Partners (1994) *Injuries at Work and Work-Related Illnesses*. Birmingham: Robin Thompson & Partners.

Tomaney, J. (1994) 'A new paradigm of work organization and technology?' in A. Amin (ed.) *Post-Fordims: A Reader*. Oxford: Blackwell.

USDAW (1992) *Work-related upper limb disorders*. Manchester: Union of Shop, Distributive and Allied Workers.

Webster, F. and Robins, K. (1993) '"I'll be watching you": comment on Sewell and Wilkinson', *Sociology*, **27**(2) May: 43–52.

Wilkin, P. (1996) 'New myths for the south: globalisation and the conflict between private power and freedom', *Third World Quarterly*, **17**(2): 227–38.

Willis, E. (1994) *Illness and Social Relations: Issues in the Sociology of Health Care*. Sydney: Allen & Unwin.

Womack, J., Roos, D. and Jones, D. (1990) *The Machine that Changed the World*. Oxford: Maxwell Macmillan International.

Wright, G.D. (1987) 'The failure of the RSI concept', *Medical Journal of Australia*, **147**: 233–6.

Wright, P. and Treacher, A. (1982) (eds) *The Problem of Medical Knowledge: Examining the Social Construction of Medicine*. Edinburgh: Edinburgh University Press.

9 ZONES OF DANGER, ZONES OF SAFETY: DISABLED PEOPLE'S NEGOTIATIONS AROUND SICKNESS AND THE SICK RECORD

Ruth Pinder

In this chapter, some of the limitations as well as the strengths of either/or dichotomies which often characterise representations of health, illness and disability are explored. Through the case studies of three individuals with impairments – not necessarily caused by the work setting – the author highlights the fluid and emergent nature of people's characterisations of themselves as they negotiate the shifting boundaries of the external world: neither health, illness nor disability is a fixed, immutable state. If employment policies and practices are to retain and capitalise on disabled people's work skills and training, new approaches are needed which embrace the ambiguities of experience rather than trying to gloss over or control them.

When I look back on it, I don't know how I coped with going in. In all honesty, I don't know why I did either because I was so terribly ill. (Elaine)[1]

I don't think the sickness record should be linked to a disability at all because if you're disabled, it doesn't necessarily mean you're going to be off sick a lot. This is a preconceived idea that a lot of employers do have. (Simone)

Disabled people shouldn't be treated in the same way that someone else who has to have, perhaps, two months off sick a year. (Emma)

Introduction

Sickness or illness is almost always disruptive and nowhere more so than in the workplace. As 'matter out of place', it is a highly charged issue. For employers, the matter is usually seen in terms of 'controlling absenteeism' (*Croner's Guide*, 1993), being primarily a question of work discipline and regulation. For the employee, questions of fault lie only partly concealed beneath the surface, and the issue of his/her genuineness is always at stake in gauging whether or not to take time off: an employee's moral competence is in doubt (Dodier, 1985; Tarasuk and Eakin, 1995).

Moreover, sickness at work blurs the boundaries between the public and the private, foregrounding the body and its language of distress in a way which is at variance with the norms of productivity and performance. Crucially, sickness absence creates an anomalous space where distinctions between 'same' and 'other' may become sharpened: it is a repository for our contemporary cultural ideas of danger.

Ambiguity and danger

The thorny question of going sick – or not – at work is particularly difficult for those with non-work-related disabilities, such as arthritis, as they try to 'make it' in the workplace. Arthritis often involves periods of pain and unwellness as well as disability, and sickness is a focal point of unease for those disabled people who are already vulnerable in the labour market. The sick record cannot be discounted in the way that those with stable conditions may be able to claim highly dependable work attendance records. However, anomalies, as Douglas (1966) notes 'are good to think with'.

How and why do such shifting spatial and social categories occur? The modernist impulse is to impose order upon the world, to search for clear-cut lines and concepts which cut through the complexity and ambiguity of everyday experience (Douglas, 1966; Perin, 1977, 1988; Sibley, 1996). To this end, every culture classifies the world into what is and what is not, who belongs and who does not. Our identities are carved out around these definitions. When people are neither quite one thing nor another, the human urge is to settle the matter unequivocally.

As Wardaugh (1996) notes, spatial boundaries are used across cultures to assert a moral order. There is a moral taint implicit in the meanings of such definitions, so that difference is not just difference, it is 'wrong' difference (Perin, 1977). We are uncomfortable bringing together phenomena which are *un*alike. Moreover, those at the margins of society's categories are often in an especially perilous position: they pick up pieces from either side of the boundaries. Even if the threat is more imaginary than real, there is always the danger that the 'other' may colonise the 'self'. As Douglas argues:

> Danger lies in transitional states, simply because transition is neither one state nor the next, it is undefinable. The person who must pass from one to another is himself in danger and emanates danger to others. (Douglas, 1966, p. 79)

The quest for clear lines and simple messages finds expression in our social institutions, reflected, for example, in employment policies that require employees to be *either* sick *or* fit, and is mirrored in the rules governing receipt of incapacity benefit: therapuetic earnings apart,[2] it is difficult for claimants to be partly well.

'Undersocialised' and 'oversocialised' perspectives: towards a rapprochement

There are two main discourses on sickness (or absenteeism) at work. Chiefly concerned with identifying predictors, and selecting appropriate measurements, the voluminous occupational health literature focuses on 'the characteristics of individual workers involved, particularly the 'normally fit' worker with specific work-related illnesses, and a selected range of environmental factors' (Quinlan, 1988). Moreover, in paying little attention to the many interlocking webs of significance in which going sick – or not – in the workplace is embedded, the tenor is overly psychologistic, quantitative and mechanistic, with a disturbing undercurrent of victim blaming. For conditions such as arthritis, occupational health studies are fuelled by worries about the hefty cost implications of work loss after the onset of disability and illness (Yelin, 1986; Yelin *et al.*, 1987; Reisine *et al.*, 1989; McIntosh, 1996).[3] The question of legitimating absence is highly problematic. Employees are fit-but-sick (Pinder, 1996).

Disability researchers and activists take a different view. In their struggle to integrate disabled people into the labour market, disability theorists have concentrated on structural factors, particularly the many practical barriers to participation in the workforce, as well as the more elusive and deeply entrenched problem of ablist 'attitudes' (Linton, 1988; Morrell, 1990; Oliver, 1990; Barnes, 1991; Oliver,

1996). If occupational health professionals are concerned to legitimate absence, disability activists struggle to validate presence: employees are sick-but-fit.

The social conditions which have surrounded disabled peoples' marginalisation from participation in the economy have demanded concise and exhaustive classification. Disability theorists have reformulated the International Classification of Impairments, Disabilities and Handicaps (ICIDH) first published in 1980 by the WHO, which attempted to provide a taxonomy of disease consequences and a basis for greater conceptual clarity in the field (Bury, 1987) in favour of a twofold distinction between impairment and disability. Disability is redefined as:

> The loss or limitation of opportunities that prevents people who have impairments from taking part in the normal life of the community on an equal level with others due to physical and social barriers (Swain et al., 1993)

For understandable reasons grounded in the desire of disability activists to reject the medical model of disability which has been a major source of oppression for disabled people, impairment tends to get less of a hearing.

However vital such a perspective is in the continuing struggle to obtain civil rights for disabled people, it tends to be an 'oversocialised' model (Williams, 1996): impairment and disability are syphoned off into separate compartments, and the many interconnecting layers of significance in which disability is embedded glossed over. The normative assumption that individuals are or should be essentially similar is problematic and ethnocentric. I have argued elsewhere (Pinder, 1995, 1996) that we cannot understand the experience of illness and disability at work without bringing the individual and the body back into the equation. The reification of 'disabling environments' is as disembodied as occupational health's concentration on problems of worker 'attitude' and discipline has neglected the social structure. Individual, social and political bodies are inextricably intertwined (Scheper-Hughes and Lock, 1987) and cannot be separated without doing violence to the reality of lived experience.[4]

With this complex tapestry in mind, this chapter takes a holistic approach. It explores how three informants, variously disabled with arthritis, tried to 'make it' at work around periods of sickness. Their narratives will illustrate how sickness and the sick record become moral sites of danger, and the chapter traces some of the consequences of this source of entrapment for the three informants concerned in the context of shifting contemporary definitions of sickness and disability. In the hope of bringing the disparate discourses of occupational health and disability closer together, the chapter briefly explores the potential of the Disability Discrimination Act 1996 to transform such classifications.

The three informants: similarities and differences

In some respects, their lives shared certain affinities. All three informants held desk jobs which, one might expect, could be more readily adapted to any impairment, and there was every indication that they were competent and hardworking in their respective jobs. Elaine was PA to the managing director of a large electronics company, Emma was a ratings assistant in her local council, and Simone PA to the chief executive of her local authority health and consumer services department.

Educationally, their attainments were comparatively modest; although all had acquired some O levels, and Emma had gained credits towards an Open University degree. Elaine became ill with rheumatoid arthritis in her mid-twenties, while both Emma and Simone had contracted juvenile chronic arthritis earlier in life, Simone in early childhood and Emma in her mid-teens. All three described themselves as 'moderately disabled' although there were wide variations in observable levels of impairment. Elaine's was barely visible, while both Emma and Simone had considerably more observable mobility and dexterity difficulties.

Their respective employment careers were different in many respects. Elaine's much loved secretarial career had been rudely terminated shortly after the onset and diagnosis of her condition. Emma had been comparatively content in post with her current employer over the past decade, when her tranquillity was abruptly disturbed by pressure to take retirement on medical grounds. By contrast, Simone's position with an equal opportunities employer was more secure, and a good working relationship with her boss allowed her to view her forthcoming hip surgery with some equanimity.

Elaine's forced exit

With the onset of rheumatoid arthritis, Elaine's close working relationship with her boss was severed. She was no longer 'his right hand and his left hand'. After a short period of sick leave to try to come to terms with the pain and fatigue which were hampering her work performance, she succumbed to the pleas of her boss, and agreed to ease her way back into work on a part-time basis in the first instance. However, the job-sharing arrangements quickly broke down, precipitating a second period of sick leave. Elaine was beginning to realise that she could no longer keep pace with the pressures of her workload. Events preceeded her. She was summoned down to the personnel office one morning and her employment was terminated with two months' salary in lieu. Her entitlement to a small pension was only discovered later after exhaustive enquiries.

Looking back, she tried to piece together the rapid escalation of events. Much centred on the intimate relationship with her boss, where small variations in mood and performance were highly visible to him, and his response to sickness:

> He had a dislike of illness... There was definite ignorance, not ignorant rude. He would not accept that I was ill. He couldn't relate, he didn't know how to react I suppose. Other people would offer compassion. He didn't understand what was happening. It needed him to say 'Elaine, you're sick, *go home*'.
>
> Everyone else could see it. I mean I was so terribly ill and I was actually walking around like this [crouched, humping her back] because I couldn't straighten my arms. Everyone else was noticing it, but he wasn't. And I can say it laughingly now, he was concerned because he wasn't getting his work done.

The lack of understanding took a particularly upsetting form, when she found the communicating door between them closed. 'As soon as I was becoming ill, and obviously I'd lost my sense of humour, that door was shut and he'd actually come through the *other* door.' It was both a physical and a symbolic marker of her altered identity and status: he could not tolerate the ambiguity of relating to a secretary who was so obviously unwell, but who continued to try and fulfil her normal 'nurturing' work.

Elaine felt that little could have been done to modify the physical or job environment to have enabled her to cope better. She was his amanuensis: 'I knew where everything was, I arranged everything: most of the job was in my head. It was a very particular position, it couldn't just be filled by temps.'

Had she 'just' been a secretary with other girls available to fill in, 'they'd have allowed me to go home and get better'. Anti-discrimination legislation, she felt, would not have made any appreciable difference:

> It wasn't a discrimination, it was practical. It was because I couldn't do the job. If I'd had the illness and could still have done the job, I'd still be there.

Seeing herself as ill rather than disabled, the services of a disability employment adviser, or local disability organisation, which might have helped her reframe her approach and explore alternative avenues for employment within the same firm, were not deemed to be relevant.

However, with time she had become more familiar with her arthritis: she knew its contours now in a way that had been little appreciated at the time.

> I can't believe now how ignorant I was at the time... If I'd got to the stage where I'm at now, that would have been different. I can cope with it now.

Events fan outwards. Now caught in a pensions trap which has effectively sealed her off from the secretarial work she loved, she felt her identity had been stripped away. The self-confidence with which she faced the world when holding down a demanding job has dwindled and she is painfully conscious of the fact that:

> I lose out on identity not being there with other people. It's made me shy. I wasn't very confident before I got the job, but I became confident. Now I'm not working, I blubber and blubber on the phone and I do dislike myself for it.

During the space of eight months, Elaine's life was turned upside down and her work identity stripped away. Although she has made adjustments since then, and is now fully occupied with cake-making and decorating classes, her new busyness cannot entirely compensate for the loss of the person she once was. Ironically, she found not long afterwards that the firm's first disabled secretary had been appointed. Perhaps her story had not been in vain after all?

Elaine's physical distress had created a difficult predicament for her boss. At one level, her new bodily rhythm was conspicuously out of step with the flow of work demanded by him (Bellaby, 1992). At a deeper level, her illness had represented a profound threat for him, severing the intimacy and privacy of their relationship. As Douglas (1966) has argued, for interaction to proceed smoothly, the body has to be 'framed out' of consciousness. Yet, pain and fatigue are particularly difficult to legitimate in the work setting (Tarasuk and Eakin, 1995). Elaine's physical distress was all too conspicuous, so that his attempts to carry on as though nothing had changed after her return from sick leave were of little avail. The situation had changed, irrevocably so, and it seemed that he could no longer trust her as the responsible and reliable PA she had been.

Emma's 'strange encounter'

If Elaine's work narrative was one of disappointed ambitions, Emma's 'awakening', although not so immediately serious in its consequences, nevertheless had a profound impact on her self-confidence.

After her discharge from residential care at the age of eighteen, Emma longed to stretch her wings. Early contact with the disability rehabilitation officer gave her a rude introduction to the culture of low expectations for disabled people in the mid-1970s. The idea of basket making in a day centre filled her with dismay. Spurred on by her parents, she had found a temporary post in the borough treasurer's department at her local council, which subsequently led to a permanent position in the ratings department. Negotiating sickness absence had not been a problem at that stage:

> If I had to go off for operations, they were quite understanding about all I'd gone through. Maybe that had something to do with the fact that these days there's more emphasis on costing everything up and getting the maximum amount of work from people for the minimum amount of pay. In local government, there used to be a lot of people employed and time off was easily covered. Nowadays, it's pared down to the bare minimum. With a disability, you're a bit of a liability sometimes. Employers are less tolerant of you having time off for things, 'cos it's going to disrupt office procedures, and they're going to have to get other people to do your work.

Remission of her condition in the 1980s – as she put it 'the disease had mostly burnt itself out so the problems were mainly mechanical' – prompted the search for financial independence in a flat of her own, and she was able to negotiate a full-time post with her employer. If she organised things carefully, she could cope with manual tasks:

> I'm obviously not at the speed that some people manage, but everyone's different. Some people might be quite quick at the keyboard, but slower at working out what to do with it. It's swings and roundabouts.

If not as intellectually stimulating as she might have wished, life was comfortable, and the good-humoured relationships she established with her work colleagues compensated for any unsatisfied ambitions.

The blow came without warning. She was summoned to see the council doctor, who informed her bluntly:

> 'I'm going to suggest that you retire on medical grounds.' She said she'd had a letter from the director of finance saying that he was worried about my performance, that because you've had time off, your colleagues have been under pressure, that was the way she put it. This was the first I'd

heard of it. It was very strange because my colleagues have never mentioned anything to me about this, and I feel sure they would, they're not the type of people who would keep things to themselves.

Puzzled and upset, Emma's encounter flew in the face of recent events where, despite major local government restructuring following the introduction of the council tax, her contract had been renewed and she had retained her grade. Returning to her desk, she was partly reassured that her colleagues felt she had been pulling her weight adequately, and that no such discussions with personnel had taken place. After intervention by her line manager, the matter was eventually dropped and Emma received a letter from the director of finance saying that the incident had been 'a misunderstanding'.

However, an uneasy question mark now hung over her future employment there:

> With all this restructuring they were trying to find ways of getting rid of people, the people that they *could* get rid of. The people that had disabilities seemed like the easy option because they could just look at your sickness record and say 'oh well, Mrs Bloggs has had sixty days off this year, so we'll try and get rid of her.' I felt this was unfair because you can't really compare *me* to someone who's one hundred per cent fit in their health. The reason I'm having to have time off is for operations to try and improve my health. If I don't have these things done, I'm going to end up not being able to work at all. They knew what I had wrong with me when they took me on. I don't think that people with disabilities who're being employed on that basis should be treated in the same way as someone who has to have, perhaps, two months off sick a year.

A profound sense of injustice informed Emma's understandings of the encounter. The interview with the council doctor had been more of an ultimatum than a negotiation. Moreover, it was an ultimatum at variance with the way she had recently been classified by her employing authority, and with the understandings she had built up over the years with her colleagues. No longer entirely trustful of her workmates, sickness had become a focal point of unease for Emma, reflected in her precise tally of '89 days' absence in October 1993' on the questionnaire which she completed prior to the interview. She had exhausted the 'fund of permissable sick leave' (Herzlich and Pierret, 1987). Even with planned absence, she evidently had little in the kitty.

Emma's story showed that the limits of tolerance were highly variable. Absence that was unremarkable in the 1970s and boom years of the 1980s was now sharply penalised in the more stringent economic climate of the 1990s. An equal opportunities policy was evidently a moveable feast.

Simone: 'It's a two-way thing dealing with employment'

If Elaine and Emma had both brushed against the sharper edge of employment disadvantage that many disabled people routinely experience, Simone's situation was brighter.

Disabled early in childhood, she had nonetheless managed to secure a fairly regular education. However, applying for her first job as a shorthand typist was still a significant hurdle to overcome. Now aged 34, armed with her parents' support, and with growing confidence in her ability to 'market' herself, she is holding down a responsible position as personal assistant to one of her local authority's directors.

She had learnt to handle tricky questions from employers about any sickness absences early on, and her health record was a source of pride. 'Apart from one period of nine months in 1983, I'm *never* off sick for more than a few days' she explained. Recalling the interview for her present post she reflected:

> At some point in the conversation I did happen to say that my general health is excellent. I haven't had much time off sick. I asked them if they wanted to know anything about my disability or the time I've had in hospital, and they said 'your general sickness looks excellent'. They actually mentioned at the interview 'we are an equal opps employer and disability is looked at differently from people who have frequent Friday afternoons off with a headache.'

A similarly determined yet flexible attitude characterised her approach to her workload. She fitted the many demands for her attention around her physical difficulties, – and her job gave her that leeway – 'batching things up instead of reacting to everything that comes along' to avoid the fatigue and pain which her impairment often caused. It had not always been so:

> I have been guilty in the past of always being the one that'll stay behind and get something finished, feeling that I had to prove myself, not getting tired or sick and being willing, not shirking the work. And then it suddenly dawned on me the more you do that, the more people will let you do that. I've learnt to say no to those things, to be a bit more assertive.

Such an approach, she felt, was invaluable in demonstrating to employers that she had carefully considered any possible problems her impairment might pose. Her boss was a high flier, uncompromising in his expectations, but Simone had learnt to speak up – 'not *too* often, but enough if things get really bad', and her assertiveness had elicited a reasonably sympathetic response. While stressing the importance of accepting responsibility for herself, she was also crucially aware that determination 'could not achieve everything for disabled people. Having equal opportunities in place is at least the right start. Given the right help you can then help yourself much more' was the cornerstone of her philosophy.

However, her impairment was intrusive at times. With surgery for her knee joints pending, her doctor had left its precise timing up to her. Reflecting on how to maintain some continuity during her absence, Simone considered:

> It will be a disruption having them done, but I don't think my employers would find it a problem, because it's something that I've always said right from the word go when I took the job on, and as I've got promoted, it's had to be reminded that I can't guarantee that I'm not going to have to have time out for other ops. I personally would want it to be as short a time as possible. But I think if I just went in one day and said to my boss 'Look, can we chat, because my knees are getting really bad, can I put myself on the waiting list?' then they would just say 'Fine: let us know when it's going to be and we'll have to make some arrangement'.

Cover which was already routinely provided when she went on annual leave could readily be adapted to periods of sickness. Moreover, Simone was considering asking her boss to install a terminal at home until she was fully recovered. The council's written conditions of employment could not have provided a starker contrast with her earlier job experience working for a pharmacist. Accounts from her friends, similarly disabled with arthritis, reminded her all too painfully of the way in which sick leave was often represented:

> Women friends of mine have been off for hysterectomies and it's been 'my God, why are they doing that to us' kind of thing. No one chooses to have these things done, but that's been the attitude. I feel a bit more secure now in being able to work round things and suggest things. It's a two-way thing dealing with employment.

Crucially what Simone referred to as 'the basics', such as accessible parking, were in place for her, allowing disabled people to flourish. Unlike Emma, rhetoric matched reality, and a vigorous equal opportunities policy was carefully adhered to by her employing organisation. In addition, knowing how to manage her body, particularly the pain and fatigue which periodically assailed her, allied to careful planning, were the hallmarks of Simone's ability to hold down a pressured job, and the promotion she had recently been awarded. Planned sick leave was acceptable, so long as she did not exhaust the fund of goodwill which she had earned. Moreover, excellent working relationships with her boss were not threatened by unpredictable flares of her illness in the way experienced by Elaine: the private world of the body was kept tolerably at bay. Despite substantial impairment, she was not being forced into early retirement on medical grounds, at least for the fore-seeable future. She inhabited a comparatively safe social space.

Discussion: zones of safety, zones of danger

After nearly 30 years of campaigning, an increasing number of disabled people are gradually being integrated into the labour market, becoming 'same' rather than 'other'. However, for two of the three informants discussed here, overstepping the limits of tolerance as far as sick leave was concerned immediately relocated disability as 'other', putting disabled people 'back in their place' as it were . While the ambiguities of a certain amount of sickness and sick leave might (variously) be tolerated, an accumulating sick record was likely to sharply differentiate self from 'other'. Sickness at work, and the sick record were sites of danger and a source of vulnerability for people with non-work-related impairments. Three areas merit further discussion.

Contested boundaries, contested identities

A picture of overlapping categories has emerged, with informants often finding themselves painfully '"betwixt and between" all the recognised fixed points in space-time classification' (Turner, 1967, p. 96). Their stories fitted neither the clear lines of the occupational health discourse nor that of mainstream disability studies with their comparative silencing of the body. Different though Elaine, Emma and Simone's stories were in detail, their stories illustrate the difficulties of confining the lived experience of arthritis at work to one discrete domain or the other.

Were they partly well, partly sick or disabled? Had the complex realities of their respective experiences been more neatly resolvable, some of the conflicts in their work situations might have been avoided.

For both Emma and Elaine, the more ambiguous the boundaries, the more dangerous – and polluting – were their attempts to occupy the liminal space in between. Their stories attest to the difficulties of entertaining 'unfamiliar combinations of familiar things' (Perin, 1988, p. 21).

Elaine, for example, was no longer fully able-bodied, yet the disabled world did not yet beckon. She saw herself primarily as ill (although at interview her perceptions were changing), so that the thought of approaching disabled support services for help in negotiating a compromise with her boss had not occurred to her. Above all, her story illustrates the moral ambiguity of being ill 'in the wrong place', and the ambiguity was only resolved by her expulsion from the workforce. As Perin (1988, p. 22) notes: 'If keeping meanings intact is self-preservative... it is all too often other-destructive'.

By contrast, Emma had attempted to reframe the sickness issue, but found that the disability discourse upon which she attempted to draw fitted only uneasily into that equation. Its messages were too sharply drawn to fit unequivocally the complexities of her situation, and, moreover, were at odds with the equally clear modernist imperative of her employing organisation to maintain an uninterrupted flow of work. She was asking for difference to be accommodated, for ambiguity to be tolerated, but difference was precisely what an overstretched local authority needed to smoothe away in the interests of a once-and-for-all narrative of completion and safety. Paradoxically, her insistence on the purity of a category – that she was not 'doing normal sickness', that disabled sickness was something apart, – added to the hazards of her predicament. Her brush with danger had almost succeeded in confirming her identity as 'different' – and undesirably so.

Simone, on the other hand, was able to cross the threshold between disability and sickness without her identity being unduly compromised – for the time being. With scrupulously husbanded sickness absence – reminiscent more of carefully planned annual leave – she could, within limits, mediate between able-bodied and disabled worlds. Seeing herself as an 'ambassador for disabled people', she occupied a potentially powerful place on the margins, able to 'play' a little with norms, rules, and established hierarchies. Rather than being negatively anomalous, her space was positively singular: she combined unfamiliar things in familiar ways. Yet mindful of the power of sickness and the sick record to circumscribe disabled people's lives, hers was a contingent work future. She was not entirely certain that she would be able to hold down a highly pressured job in the longer term.

Webs of significance

As Bellaby (1989) makes clear 'what constitutes acceptable absence from work or not is secured by the evolution of conventions which are themselves framed by fellow employees, employers, medical practitioners, and close relatives in the context of particular economic and historical circumstances.' Taking time off, he concludes:

> is a structured social process which is reducible neither to morbidity nor to individual reasoning in isolation from other people and from conventions of conduct. (1989, p. 424)

With only modest educational qualifications apiece, all three informants found themselves caught in wider structural constraints which limited their ability to manoeuvre. As female white-collar workers, they occupied a comparatively weak bargaining position in the labour market, regardless of illness and disability. Elaine's illness sharpened inequalities which were already well entrenched. As Putnam and Mumby (1993:46) note 'sexuality and emotional bonding are basic to the practices which constitute secretaries as objects' – and the emotional nurturing provided in secretary–boss relationships is usually expendable.

Neither can Emma and Simone's positions be understood without reference to the major structural upheavals occurring in local government in the late 1980s and early 1990s. Emma found herself caught in the contradictions between rhetoric and reality: between the ethos of an organisation which officially endorsed an equal opportunities policy and the harsh realities of downsizing and cost-cutting exercises required by local authorities in an economy only barely emerging from recession. In the contemporary economic climate of heightened job insecurity, anxieties about maintaining existing body boundaries and body purity were exacerbated.

The disparity between rhetoric and reality were less marked for Simone in the more affluent Home Counties. Moreover, while she was unequivocal about the vital importance of providing 'the basics' for disabled people in the workplace, her strong sense of responsibility and refusal to see 'society' as entirely to blame for the exclusion of disabled people from mainstream society (see Hillyer, 1993, p. 112, on this point) articulated well with the logic of enterprise which characterised her working partnership (Keat and Abercrombie, 1991). Her particular strength lay in the ability to move between the discourse of self-actualisation and individual responsibility, and the trenchant critique of modernity and neo-liberalism provided by the Disability Movement.

The sick record and the social control of space

The three informants' stories not only represent an attempt to redefine and secure shifting definitions of sickness, illness and disability, they also illustrate attempts to regulate and discipline those who inhabit such dangerous social margins within the labour market. Sickness and the sick record were the pivots around which judgements about their moral competence and effective membership of the workforce – or not – hung. Emma's '89 days' for example, was not only an 'objective' tally of days lost; it was also a symbolic marker, where her genuineness and credibility were in question. Similarly, the pensions trap in which Elaine now found herself constrained her future possibilities in a way quite unanticipated by her initial sickness. And Simone, knowing how easily sickness could become a source of entrapment for disabled people, was appropriately wary of it.

Foucault has alerted us to the way in which records represent:

> the fixing, at once ritual and 'scientific' of individual difference… [they are] a process by which an individual is linked by his status to the features, the measurements, the gaps, the 'marks' that characterise him [sic] and make him a 'case'. (1977, p. 1996)

From criminal dossiers to 'the fat envelope patient', records acquire a facticity often more real than the lives of those whose characteristics they purport to encapsulate. The sick record acted as a shorthand for Emma's medical condition, glossing over the many relevant non-phys-ical aspects of her life. A key site of vulnerability for disabled people, it regulated connections between fitness and sickness, safety and danger in the workplace, functioning as a 'discourse which uses the "other" as a "useful" source of danger' (Carter, 1996, p. 145). As Frankenberg (1992) points out: 'Those groups facing danger which can be defined as "other" often face controls which work in the interests of the powerful "same"'.

A way forward?

These narratives were gathered before the Disability Discrimination Act, which made it unlawful to discriminate in the field of employment and which outlaws discrimination in the provision of goods and services and the letting of premises, came into force in December 1996. It is fair to assume that had the legislation been in place, the harshness of Elaine's sentence might have been tempered, and Emma's 'strange encounter' handled with more sensitivity and circumspection.

For disabled people in Britain, the Act is a disappointing compromise, and the challenge is now to secure much broader civil rights legislation which is both comprehensive and enforceable, on a par with the Americans with Disabilities Act 1990. Disability theorists have painted a less than optimistic picture of the extent to which disabled people are likely to penetrate the labour market (Oliver, 1990).

Both Doyle (1995) and Abberley (1996, p. 71), have commented on 'the romanticism of productivity', fearing that any softening of society's stance is likely to sharpen the divisions between 'acceptably' disabled workers and the remainder. New boundaries and new zones of safety and danger will be created.

Those reservations apart, the picture may not be quite so bleak. The Act is still the most significant anti-discrimination legislation of recent years and 'change by stealth' may be a powerful – if underrated – transformative force. Taking a leaf from education, change often only 'takes' if it is 'nearly new' and embedded in structures which are already familiar and well established. Even though the more intangible aspects of relationships between able-bodied and disabled people may still prove to be more refractory, shifting classifications, however imperfect, give reasonable grounds for cautious optimism.

One of the tasks of this chapter has been to illustrate the dangers of viewing definitions of sickness, illness and disability as fixed and immutable. To do so implies a certain false coherence, uniformity and timelessness to the meanings of sickness and sickness absence at work. What has emerged most powerfully from the three informants' accounts is the shifting, fluid nature of those classifications of the self and other. Boundaries are constantly being fashioned and refashioned in response to the many changing social, economic and cultural currents which form the backcloth to disabled people's lives: 'Process is what happens all the time' (Bohannan, 1995). Professor Williams' provocative thoughts on racism in the 1997 Reith Lectures have alerted us to the fact that complex differences have to be continually negotiated.

The conductor Daniel Barenboim has often urged aspiring musicians to pay attention to the space between the notes as much as to the notes themselves. Similarly, this chapter has alerted us to the importance of looking at the spaces between categories, to the many linkages which bind people with disabilities to the wider world, so that we may move more fluently between able-bodied (or temporarily able-bodied as Irving Zola once quipped) and disabled worlds. It is hoped that the three informants' narratives presented here may alert us to the ways in which disability and illness, sickness and the sick record, are more readily identifiable as part of our problem, rather than being seen as repositories of danger and uncertainty.

Notes

1   These are not their real names: I have used pseudonyms throughout. The three informants' narratives presented here formed part of a wider qualitative research project part funded by *Arthritis Care*, 1993–1994, and I gratefully acknowledge their support.

2   Social security regulations state that claimants are able to earn a small sum each week in work if such work is deemed to be of a therapeutic nature. In practice, it has become too risky for most disabled people to lodge such a claim, as one's incapacity for work is immediately suspect.

3   McIntosh (1996) found, for example, that the total economic impact of rheumatoid arthritis in the UK in 1992 was estimated to be £1.26 billion, 'of which 52 per cent was a result of lost production'.

4   The social model is now being vigorously debated by disabled people within the Disability Movement, and a wider definition may be forthcoming.

Bibliography

Abberley, P. (1996) 'Work, Utopia and impairment' in L. Barton (ed.) *Disability and Society: Emerging Issues and Insights*. Harlow: Addison Wesley Longman.

Barnes, C. (1991) *Disabled People in Britain and Discrimination: A Case for Anti-Discrimination Legislation*. London: Hurst.

Bellaby, P. (1989) 'The social meanings of time off work: a case study from a pottery factory', *Annals of Occupational Hygiene*, **33**(3): 423–38.

Bellaby, P. (1990) 'What is genuine sickness? The relation between work-discipline and the sick role in a pottery factory', *Sociology of Health and Illness*, **12**(1): 47–68.

Bellaby, P. (1992) 'Broken rhythms and unmet deadlines' in R. Frankenberg (ed.), *Time, Health and Medicine*. London: Sage.

Bohannan, P. (1995) *How Culture Works*. New York: Free Press.

Bury, M. (1987) 'The ICIDH: a review of research and prospects', *Intl Disability Studies*, **9**: 118–28.

Carter, S. (1995) 'Boundaries of danger and uncertainty: an analysis of the technological culture of risk assessment' in J. Gabe (ed.), *Medicine, Health and Risk: Sociological Approaches*. Oxford: Blackwell.

Croner's Guide to Managing Absence (1993) (3rd edn). Surrey: Croner.

Department of Social Security (1989) *Employers' Manual of Statutory Sick Pay*, No. 0800 393539.

Dodier, N. (1985) 'Social uses of illness at the workplace: sick leave and moral evaluation', *Social Science and Medicine*, **20**(2): 123–8.

Douglas, M. (1966) *Purity and Danger: An Analysis of the Concepts of Pollution and Taboo*. London: Routledge.

Doyle, B. (1995) Disability, Discrimination and Equal Opportunities: *A Comparative Study of Employment Rights of Disabled People*. London: Mansell.

Foucault, M. (1977) *Discipline and Punish: The Birth of the Prison*. Harmondsworth: Penguin.

Frankenberg, R. (1992) 'The "other" who is also the "same": the relevance of epidemics in space and time for the prevention of HIV infection', *International Journal of Health Services*, **22**(1): 73–88.

French, S. and Finkelstein, V. (1993), 'Towards a psychology of disability' in J. Swain, V. Finkelstein, S. French and M. Oliver (eds), *Disabling Barriers and Enabling Environments*. London: Sage.

Goodman, P.S. and Atkin, R.S. (1984) *Absenteeism: New Approaches to Measuring and Managing Employee Absence*. San Francisco: Jossey-Bass.

Herzlich, C. and Pierret, J. (1987) *Illness, Self and Society*. London: Johns Hopkins.

Hillyer, B. (1993) *Feminism and Disability*. Norman: University of Oklahoma Press.

Keat, R. and Abercrombie, N. (eds) (1991) *Enterprise Culture*. London: Routledge.

Linton, S. (1998) *Claiming Disability: Knowledge and Identity*. New York: New York University Press.

McIntosh, E. (1996) 'The cost of rheumatoid arthritis', *British Journal of Rheumatology*, **35**: 781–90.

Morrell, J. (1990) *The Employment of People with Disabilities: Research into the Policies and Practices of Employers*. London: IFF Research.

Oliver, M. (1990) *The Politics of Disablement*. Basingstoke: Macmillan.

Oliver, M. (1996) *Understanding Disability: From Theory to Practice*. Basingstoke: Macmillan.

Perin, C. (1977) *Everything in its Place: Social Order and Land Use in America*. New Jersey: Princeton University Press.

Perin, C. (1988) *Belonging in America: Reading Between the Lines*. London: University of Wisconsin Press.

Pinder, R. (1995) 'Bringing back the body without the blame: the experience of ill and disabled people at work', *Sociology of Health and Illness*, **17**(5): 605–31.

Pinder, R. (1996) 'Sick-but-fit or fit-but-sick? Ambiguity and identity at the workplace' in E. Barnes and G. Mercer (eds), *Exploring the Divide: Illness and Disability*. Leeds: The Disability Press.

Putnam, L.L. and Mumby, D.K. (1993) 'Organisations, emotion and the myth of rationality' in S. Fineman (ed.), *Emotion in Organisations*. London: Sage.

Quinlan, M. (1988) 'Psychological and sociological approaches to the study of occupational illness: a critical review', *Australian and New Zealand Journal of Sociology*, **24**(2): 189–207.

Reisine, S.T., Grady, K.E., Goodenow, C. and Fifield, J. (1989) 'Work disability among women with rheumatoid arthritis', *Arthritis and Rheumatism*, **32**: 538–43.

Scheper-Hughes, N. and Lock, M. (1987) 'The mindful body: a prolegomenon to future work in medical anthropology' *Medical Anthropology Quarterly*, **1**: 6–41.

Shakespeare, T. (ed.) (1998) *The Disability Reader: Social Science Perspectives*. London: Cassel.

Sibley, D. (1996) *Geographies of Exclusion: Society and Difference in the West*. London: Routledge.

Swain, J., Finkelstein, V., French, S. and Oliver, M. (1993) *Disability Barriers – Enabling Environments*. London: Sage.

Tarasuk, V. and Eakin, J. (1995) 'The problem of legitimacy in the experience of work-related back injury', *Qualitative Health Research*, **5**(2): 204–21.

Thomas, A. (1992) *Working with a Disability: Barriers and Facilitators*. London: SPCR.

Turner, V. (1967) *The Forest of Symbols: Aspects of Ndembu Ritual*. London: Cornell University Press.

Wardaugh, J. (1996) 'Homeless in Chinatown: deviance and social control in Cardboard City', *Sociology*, **30**(4): 701–16.

Williams, G. (1996) 'Representing disability: some questions of phenomenology and politics' in C. Barnes and G. Mercer (eds), *Exploring the Divide: Illness and Disability*. Leeds: The Disability Press.

Williams, P. (1997) *The Reith Lectures*, BBC.

Yelin, E. (1986) 'The myth of malingering: why individuals withdraw from work in the presence of illness', *The Milbank Memorial Fund*, **64**(4): 622–49.

Yelin, E., Henke, C. and Epstein, W. (1987) 'The work dynamics of the person with rheumatoid arthritis', *Arthritis and Rheumatism*, **30**: 507–12.

10 Selling Sex, Giving Care: The Construction of AIDS as a Workplace Hazard

Tamsin Wilton

It is frequently assumed that the expansion of occupational health and safety provisions to all workers is a 'good thing'. This chapter challenges that view, raising important questions about the wider discourses employed to analyse and interpret HIV/AIDS risks in the workplace. The examples of care work and sex work are used to explore the different ways in which these risks are constructed depending on who is doing the defining and whose risks are being defined. In the case of sex work in particular, its status as a 'non-occupation' and the moral opprobrium attached to those who carry it out, have led to increased risk of HIV infection among what is often a particularly disadvantaged group of women. The implications of this for mainstream health and safety, health promotion and HIV/AIDS work requires careful consideration and critical reflection on current practices.

This chapter examines how AIDS-related risk has been constructed in the context of sex work and care work and, in so doing, touches on some key questions about 'occupational health': What is an occupation? What is meant by work? What is a workplace? Whose work-related health is prioritised and whose neglected? What wider sociopolitical trajectories cut across the fields of health promotion and occupational health?

The critique outlined in this chapter contributes to the development of three current critical projects; the growing awareness of the social control element present in all health and social care policy and practice (for example Gilman, 1995; Lupton, 1995; Waldby, 1996), the critical analysis of health education/promotion as a *discourse* which plays an active part in the construction of hegemonic beliefs and perceptions (for example Treichler, 1988; essays in Boffin and Gupta, 1990; Wilton, 1997), and a more general postmodern exposure of *all* the professions as political institutions engaged in struggles over hegemony (for example essays in Terry and Urla, 1995; Turner, 1995). Ironically, this (broadly postmodern) approach poses a specific problem, as highlighted by Nicholas Fox, drawing on the insights of Foucault in relation to the medical 'gaze':

> The gaze (which, as its name implies, entails the making visible of a person or a population) is a technology of power, by which the object of the gaze becomes known to the observer. This knowledge, codified and organized, becomes a resource by which the observer develops both an expertise, and a control over those s/he observes. (Fox, 1993, p. 24)

This link between observation and control obliges me explicitly to state that, in what follows, I am *not* advocating that authoritative and/or professional attention be paid to care work and sex work (already characterised by specific forms of social and cultural control) in order to subject them to the surveillant gaze of medico-legal power. There are, however, certain medico-legal rights (such as the right to seek compensation for occupational injury) which would probably benefit those engaged in such work. This is a contradiction that remains unresolved throughout the chapter and is the subject of continuing debate in the sex industry and among informal carers.

Moreover, the social and cultural arena of the erotic, of what we loosely refer to as 'sexual behaviour', has long been a particularly important site for social control, specifically in the Foucauldian sense of the exercise of disciplinary power (Foucault, 1979; Fox, 1993), and HIV/AIDS health promotion is exemplary of this. As Deborah Lupton summarizes (1995, p. 87): 'Since the advent of the HIV/AIDS epidemic, sexual behaviour has been colonized by the discourse of risk'. It is not my intention to expand this colonization of sexual behaviour.

Nor am I here using care work and sex work as 'case studies' to suggest that these are areas of work which necessarily require the establishment of a formal occupational health care infrastructure. Rather, caring and sex work are of interest as social and cultural locations *outside* generally accepted notions of what constitutes an occupation. From these two specific locations it is possible to look critically at 'occupational health' not as a professional field informed by existing notions of risk, work, entitlement and protection, but as a discourse that actively constructs such notions. The fact that it may construct as much by its silences and lack of attention to some areas as by what it says and does is a familiar concept to cultural theorists, although perhaps less familiar to those in other fields, and is one of the key elements in what follows.

A risk by any other name?

The notion of risk is central to three intersecting professional discourses which concern AIDS in the context of the workplace: health promotion, occupational health and HIV/AIDS prevention. Yet all three discourses construct workplace HIV 'risk' in different and mutually contradictory ways, and this set of differences and contradictions has important consequences both for practice within these professional spheres and hence (presumably) for the HIV-related health and safety of those individuals and groups for whom HIV/AIDS represents a work-related risk.

Within health promotion discourse (and practice) the workplace is seen as an already formalised environment that potentially offers a useful site of health educational intervention:

> Health educators have long recognised that employers have an almost unique degree of access to the adult population. Many employers have acknowledged that this access, coupled with their legal obligations and sometimes a tradition of concern for their employees' well being throws onto them some responsibility for health promotion. (Hussey, 1996, Section 5ii)

In the context of HIV infection then, the workplace is regarded as a useful environment within which health educators may target a captive audience with a range of interventions, among which might (or might not) be campaigns focusing on HIV and AIDS.

In current AIDS-related occupational health discourse, on the other hand, the 'risk' of HIV transmission in the course of work-related activity is represented as unlikely or downright unfeasible (Richardson, 1989; Goss and Adam-Smith, 1996; Hussey, 1996). Typically confident statements include: 'employees or clients with the virus do not pose a threat within the workplace' (Goss and Adam-Smith, 1996, p. 77) and 'there is no real risk of workplace transmission' (Hussey, 1996, Section 5ii). Although health care workers and, to a lesser extent, social care workers, are generally understood to be a 'special case', more at risk than other occupational groups for workplace HIV transmission, occupational health guidelines insist – and have always insisted – that the unfailing adoption of *universal precautions*[1] 'many of which are not new and should always have been applied' (Berer, 1993, p. 68), affords adequate protection (CDC, 1985; DeVita *et al.*, 1988; Manchester AIDSLINE Women's Group, n.d.). Indeed, the tendency has always been for HIV risk in health care settings to be seen as directed outwardly from the profession to its client group. There has been far more public anxiety about HIV+ health care staff infecting patients than vice versa (for example, Boseley, 1997). Within this context, AIDS is presented almost as a non-issue.

The hybrid specialism of HIV/AIDS prevention is different yet again, in that it represents AIDS as very much a workplace issue. Within the terms of this discourse, however, it is not the work-related risk of HIV transmission that is of concern. Rather, there is a recognition of the stigmatised nature of HIV and of its association with the stigmatised sexuality of gay men. This both develops out of and in turn leads to, a focus on the importance of AIDS awareness within workplaces, with the stated objective of protecting the health and safety at work of people with HIV and/or AIDS and their partners and family members. As Goss and Adam-Smith assert (1996, pp. 80–1), an 'ordinary illness' approach to HIV infection is inadequate, since it fails to take account of the wider social implications of AIDS:

> Even though [an employer's AIDS] policy may offer protection against discrimination on the grounds of HIV infection, this alone may be insufficient to deal with the ways in which the fear of AIDS can 'spill-over' (or be maliciously manipulated) into the fear of social identities.

Issues which Goss and Adam-Smith identify as significant in attempting to protect employees' health and safety against this 'spill-over' effect include homophobia, discriminatory policies for compassionate and bereavement leave and the lack of employment protection for lesbian and gay workers.

This (well founded and laudable) concern for the wider wellbeing of individuals infected or affected by HIV informs the dominant approach of AIDS organisations to workplace health and safety issues. In Britain this approach is exemplified by the National AIDS Trust's (NAT)

Companies Act! business charter initiative, a successful and innovative programme of AIDS awareness focusing on the business community and actively supported by many big players in the British business scene including WH Smith, The Body Shop, Marks & Spencer, IBM, Levi Strauss UK and over 30 other companies and public bodies. In the 1996 review of *Companies Act!*, Julian Hussey identifies workplace harassment as the overriding concern:

> If it was the danger or risk involved in AIDS that engaged the popular imagination, it was the ensuing harassment and persecution of those with HIV and AIDS that provided the real challenge to any employment campaign... the key action would be a public commitment to combat employment related discrimination on the grounds of HIV and AIDS. (Hussey, 1996, Section 4)

NAT too recognises that 'Prejudice against people with HIV and AIDS is often hard to distinguish from prejudice against gay or bisexual men' (Hussey, 1996, Section 5ii), and that measures to combat homophobia are central to the health and safety of people with HIV or AIDS in the workplace. Interestingly, NAT also regards health care workers as a special case, since although 'there is no real risk of workplace transmission' for most workers, this confidence is less absolute in a health care environment. 'Health care professionals', the report recognises, 'may sometimes face a real risk of infection if the appropriate procedures are deliberately or accidentally breached' (Hussey, 1996, Section 5v).

It is clear that 'risk' in the context of AIDS and the workplace carries fluid, unstable and shifting meanings depending on who is speaking and which group is the object of concern. The 'risks' associated with AIDS-as-occupational-hazard are multiple and include the risk of HIV transmission, the risk of homophobic or other bias-related discrimination and the risk of 'breaching' health and safety precautions. Moreover, the notion of risk appears to shift according to *which* 'workplace' is being discussed. This is the case even when the 'risky' activities remain constant. For example, activities involved in caring for people with HIV infection and/or AIDS are generally represented as requiring fewer precautions when carried out by an unpaid carer in the domestic environment than when identical activities are carried out by paid carers in a formal health care environment (for example, compare Richardson, 1989, with Centers for Disease Control, 1985). Indeed, the very notion of the 'workplace' becomes strikingly unstable in the context of AIDS.

All work and no pay makes some work 'women's work'

Caring and sex work are characterised by a complex and overdetermined association with AIDS 'risk'. Both straddle the boundary between work and not-work in a way which exposes the fragility of that boundary and troubles our easy assumption that there is such as thing as 'occupational health'. Moreover, long-standing sociocultural constructs of gender are profoundly implicated in the continuing segregation of work and not-work as we shall see. The traditional divisions between home and workplace, between the public world of commercial economic exchange and the private, intimate world of love and kinship, are maintained with a demonstrable degree of anxiety and at a very real cost. That cost includes the inability of large numbers of women to protect themselves against a range of occupation-related harms, including the possibility of HIV infection.

Feminist researchers have amassed a considerable body of evidence about the complex relationship between dominant discourses of gender – what it means to be a 'proper' woman or a 'proper' man – and of work (for example, Cockburn, 1983, 1985, 1987a, b; Martin, 1987; Adkins, 1995). In terms of occupation-related HIV risk, Emily Martin's work is of particular interest.

For love or money? Digging up the root of all evil

Researching how women experience female bodily events such as menstruation and menopause, Martin presents a highly persuasive model of the workplace as a social location where the failure to meet women's biological needs (in the form of inadequate restroom facilities and so on) expresses a general *hostility* to the very presence of women's bodies in the work environment (see also Cockburn, 1983, 1985, 1987b). Her focus is on the cultural meanings ascribed to female reproductivity, rather than on a sociology of work or of workplace health, so that she does not fully develop these arguments. Nevertheless, her insights do offer a useful position from which to analyse the sociocultural aspects of gendered work, and the (currently invisible) implications of these for occupational health and for gendered notions of workplace 'risk'. Martin suggests that a continuing binary division of contemporary industrial societies into public/private must be understood as gendered:

> Our lives have come to be organized around two realms: a private realm where women are most in evidence, where 'natural' functions like sex... take place, where the affective content of relationships is primary, and a public realm where men are most in evidence, where 'culture'... is produced, where money is made, work is done, and where one's efficiency at producing goods or services takes precedence over one's feelings about fellow workers. (Martin, 1987, pp. 15–16)

One of the innovative features of this model is Martin's emphasis on *emotion*, which, although it has been discussed by some feminist social scientists (for example, Doyal, 1995), continues to be ignored within both mainstream social science[2] and occupational health. Yet there is an argument for recognising emotion not simply as a *marker* for the familiar social divide into public and private spheres, but as one of the primary *definitional* categories from which many of the key binary structures of modern capitalist societies develop. As long ago as 1969, David Schneider suggested that:

> The contrast between love and money... stands for home and work. Indeed, what one does at home, it is said, one does for love, not for money, while what one does at work one does strictly for money, not for love... Where love is spiritual, money is transient and contingent. (cited in Martin, 1987, p. 17)

This points to a culturally and socially hegemonic system of value and meaning which is organised not so much around a public/private split, but rather around a boundary which sets a *commercial* arena (where money is the medium of exchange) firmly apart from an *emotional* arena (whose currency is love). Moreover, as Martin recognises, these two arenas are gendered, so that commerce is regarded as the proper business of men (and widely regarded as 'work'), while emotion is regarded as the proper business of women and is marked by a constant struggle to define it as work (Martin, 1987; Malos, 1996). And indeed, the literature on HIV risk in the context of caring and prostitution is characterised not simply by a *failure* to regard these activities as work, but by a *resistance* to so doing. Yet, as we shall see, it is precisely because they are located at the definitional boundary between emotion and commerce (private/public, home/work, female/male) that carers and (especially) prostitutes are potentially at risk from HIV infection. Moreover, the '"official" response for HIV/AIDS' has been fixed within the framework of 'a medico-legal-economic alliance' (Goss and Adam-Smith, 1996, p. 79). It is difficult to see how it could make sense of the work-related needs of these groups.

Can't buy me love?

Both sex work and care work take their sociocultural meaning from their position in relation to the emotion/commerce boundary. Because caring has been naturalised as something intrinsic to being female, and because the values it carries are the domestic, familial ones of nurturance, intimacy and love, there is a cultural resistance to 'commercialising' it. Thus family and friends, and those who do it for strangers on a charitable basis, are expected to do it for free while those who do it professionally are expected to do it for low wages. As feminist commentators have pointed out, this ideological refusal to allow commercial interest to 'taint' the emotional work of caring results in the wholesale exploitation of women's labour (Land, 1991; Graham, 1993; Doyal, 1995).

On the other hand, since sex is supposed to be inextricably tied both to emotion (love, desire, intimacy, jealousy and so on) and to the family (both because heterosex is sanctioned by marriage and because it is naturalised as *for the purposes of* reproduction and pair bonding), it too is positioned firmly on the 'emotion' side of the emotion/commerce boundary. You are not supposed to pay for sex, nor to charge for it. Indeed, it is the *commercial*, rather than the *sexual* nature of the transaction which is explicitly identified as what is 'wrong', morally, with prostitution. Carole Pateman (1988, p. 196) cites the report of the Royal Commission into the Sexual Offences Act:

> There is no comparison to be made between prostitutes and the men who consort with them. With the one sex, the offence is committed as a matter of gain; with the other, it is an irregular indulgence of a natural impulse.

Of course this official statement – assuming in its innocence that all prostitutes are female and (probably with better reason) that all clients of prostitutes are male – classically demonstrates the sexual double standard. It also suggests that erasing the distinction between emotion and commerce provokes tremendous anxiety (Hobson, 1987; Treichler, 1988). Although the risks involved in both sex work and caring work are related to the location of both occupations on the emotion/commerce boundary, they are positioned as polar opposites across that boundary line, and will be discussed separately.

'You cannot catch AIDS by loving, caring and sharing'[3]

The nature and degree of occupational HIV risk for carers is influenced by the context in which they work. Caring for a person with HIV/AIDS

(PWHA) in the domestic environment almost always means working with a single individual, often a partner but overwhelmingly an adult child (Panos, 1990), for a fixed and relatively short period of time. The typical scenario is that the adult child returns to the parental home in the late stages of physical deterioration, to be cared for during the remaining months before death (Dowling, 1994). Caring for PWHAs in the voluntary sector may mean training as a 'buddy',[4] and providing care to a series of individual PWHAs in their own home, usually until their death. Care work in the statutory sector, although it may be quite intensively one to one, generally involves working with much larger numbers of individuals during short periods when they are in hospital or in the community. However, the health risks relating to these different scenarios are very similar.

Caring for PWHAs involves negligible risk of HIV infection for the carer, although even in the domestic sector those doing such work are often required to carry out surprisingly technical procedures such as changing IVs or helping with Hickman lines (Richardson, 1989), as well as handling faeces, urine, vomit, sputum or blood. The most risky care-related activities are those involving contaminated sharps, but the risk of acquiring infection through needlestick is now known to be very remote (Richardson, 1989). Other potential risks are likely to include musculoskeletal injuries from incorrect lifting techniques, exhaustion, anxiety, depression and stress-related illnesses (Wilson, 1993; Dowling, 1994). To a great extent, the occupational risks associated with caring for PWHAs are those of care work generally, since carers tend to be 'a group who have poorer physical and emotional health than non-carers' (Galbally, 1997, p. 17).

Although such risks are routinely addressed in the nursing literature, they are notably absent from literature either discussing or addressing those caring for PWHAs outside the formal sector. Clearly, risks that are labelled 'occupational health hazards' within the commercial arena are not recognised as such when they are encountered elsewhere. Voluntary and informal caring are not 'occupations', therefore the health hazards associated with them are not 'occupational'. It must be concluded that occupational health discourse[5] *constructs* non-commercial care work as a non-occupation.

Bridgeheads and foul sewers: anything but work

In contrast to the relatively simple failure of occupational health to recognise unpaid care work, prostitution is subject to an altogether more complex and sinister treatment. It is not the case that prostitutes have been ignored in AIDS prevention. Indeed, they have arguably been more widely studied in the interests of AIDS prevention than any other sexual cohort with the possible exception of gay men (Whittaker and Hart, 1996). This research activity has not, however, generally been motivated by a concern for sex workers' health.

Euroamerican cultures share a shameful history of prostitute-blaming, holding them responsible for everything from the fall of empires to the spread of venereal disease (Wells, 1982; Hobson, 1987; Treichler, 1988; Wilton, 1997).[6] This unpleasant tradition has been carried on in the context of AIDS, where prostitutes are seen as reservoirs of infection waiting to infect their clients (Treichler, 1988; Patton, 1994; Wilton, 1997), and where 'advice to men about using condoms centers almost exclusively on the risk *to them* of sex for payment' (Patton, 1994, p. 109, added emphasis). Scambler and Scambler (1995 and this volume) point to 'the paradox that the rational and often innovative work now being done... oriented to improving the health status and prospects of women sex workers... has been made possible by "AIDS money" generated in part through moral panic' (Scambler and Scambler, 1995, p. 17)

There is an extensive literature on prostitution in the broad field of health studies. Within this literature, prostitution is described as many things, but seldom as an occupation. It has been described as a pathology, a disorder of sexual function (Wells, 1982; Hobson, 1987), a form of or consequence of intellectual impairment (Wells, 1987), a criminal activity (Barnard and McKeganey, 1996), or a form of immorality (Brandt, 1987; Hobson, 1987). Prostitutes have been described as 'foul sewers' (Wells, 1982, p. 65), 'seminal drains' (Treichler, 1988, p. 262) or bridgeheads of HIV infection (Barnard and McKeganey, 1996). Particularly notable is the insistence of many AIDS researchers on regarding sex work as a *sexual*, rather than a *commercial* encounter[7] – and consequently sex workers themselves as sexually promiscuous individuals, rather than a segment of the labour force enduring appalling working conditions (for example, Kilpatrick and Kilpatrick, 1987).

Those researchers who do treat prostitution as work are generally those who have a more sympathetic and sensitive attitude to their research subjects, and their research demonstrably yields more detailed and useful findings with regard not only to AIDS prevention, but to general issues of occupational health for sex workers (Venema and Visser, 1990; Bloor *et al.*, 1991; Scambler and Scambler, 1995; Barnard and McKeganey, 1996; Pyett and Warr, 1996, 1997; Whittaker and Hart, 1996). Nevertheless, almost without exception these researchers are at pains to stress how *different* prostitution is from other forms of work. This difference is identified as arising from the illegitimate and criminal status of sex work (in most countries) and its associated stigma (Leonard and Thistlethwaite, 1990; Barnard and McKeganey, 1996; Pyett and Warr, 1996).

As with care work, sex work takes place in a range of different environments and exposure to occupational hazards is related to these. The callgirl operating from a flat with the assistance of a 'maid', the woman working in a brothel or massage parlour, the rent boy picking up in local public toilets or cruising site, the street walker plying for hire on street corners and the unstructured encounters of the drug addict selling sex in response to the demands of her habit are all exposed to risk of different kinds and in different degrees. As Priscilla Pyett and Deborah Warr (1996, p. 7) typically conclude: 'It was expected that different modes of sex work (that is, street, brothel, escort or private) would determine the extent to which women's physical safety was endangered, and this was borne out by our data.'

It is recognised that women engaged in sex work are at increased risk of cervical cancer, genital inflammations and infections and sexually transmitted diseases (including HIV) simply because of the frequency with which they have intercourse, and these risks are increasingly perceived as occupational hazards, at least by some researchers (Messing *et al.*, 1993; Pyett and Warr, 1996, 1997). However, recent research also indicates that there are multiple health consequences relating to the stigmatised and criminalised nature of their occupation. For example, Pyett and Warr (1996) identified stress, depression, problems with pregnancy, sleep disturbance, social isolation and hepatitis, as well as HIV infection, as occupational health hazards of the women they interviewed. Most surveys agree that violence is an ever present threat to women sex workers (Venema and Visser, 1990; Karim *et al.*, 1993; Barnard and McKeganey, 1996; Whittaker and Hart, 1996), and Pyett and Warr are typical in finding that: 'A number of women felt that because they were a prostitute there was little point in seeking legal redress if they were assaulted or raped by clients' (1996, p. 8).

Moreover, the location of sex work outside the structures of the formal labour market compromises the health of its workforce in other ways, especially in countries such as the USA where there is no national health service. 'Because prostitution is illegal, employers are not responsible to sex workers in any way. Sex workers have no job-related health or disability benefits, making health care difficult to obtain' (Leonard and Thistlethwaite, 1990, p. 181). This has clear implications for HIV-related occupational health, both within an HIV/AIDS prevention framework and within a traditional workplace-based occupational health model.

There is one area where immediate benefits could be gained by recognising the HIV-associated risks of sex work as occupational health issues, and that is in the legalistic context of tort and compensation. If health care professionals become HIV infected in the course of their work, they may have recourse to some form of compensation, and may draw on the resources of trades unions, professional bodies or legal advisors to help them do so. While it is clearly inadequate to think in terms of setting a price on illness and death, such compensation is of particular benefit in countries, such as the USA, where health care is a commercial enterprise. Yet, as Zoe Leonard and Polly Thistlethwaite comment: 'Just imagine the possibility of a prostitute charging a john with infecting her!' (1990 p. 182).

One key issue which distinguishes prostitution from most other occupations is its complex legal status which plays a part in maintaining its position as a marginal, deviant behaviour rather than an accepted occupation. Because criminalisation is associated with specific occupational hazards for sex workers, there is a strong health promotional argument in favour of decriminalisation. Where prostitution is decriminalised, working conditions are greatly improved, and the health and safety aspects of sex work become identified and addressed. Holland decriminalised prostitution for this reason and, as Venema and Visser report (1990), this has brought very real benefits in terms of protecting the physical safety of the workforce, offering employment protection to brothel workers and facilitating measures to protect both workers and consumers from HIV and other STDs. In Australia, the state of Victoria has also decriminalised sex work in the context of registered brothels, and here too the legislative change has resulted in very real improvement in working conditions. Brothels in Victoria offer a real degree of physical safety, support for the workers to insist on condom use, and the security of a structured work environment. Moreover:

> the Prostitution Control Act... demonstrates the community's acceptance of prostitution as a legitimate business. Women working as prostitutes are therefore entitled to the same level of support and protection for their occupational health as any other member of the community. (Pyett and Warr, 1996, p. 22)

Given the complexities of the cultural and juridical construction of prostitution as a non-occupation, it is unclear whether decriminalisation on its own would be sufficient to recast it as a job like any other. Nor is this necessarily desirable. However, decriminalisation can offer important protection to those workers who choose or are able to work within its limits. Moreover, Pyett and Warr suggest that some indirect benefits may accrue to those women who, through choice or necessity, continue to work outside the legitimised brothels,[8] since it might 'help to reduce the stigma attached to sex work which currently contributes to women's low self-esteem and their acceptance of violence as a condition of being engaged in prostitution' (1996, p. 21).

However, it is not only the illegality of sex work that makes it so 'different' from other occupations and leads to specific health risks, particularly in the context of HIV. As Barnard and McKeganey (1996) recognise, the fact that prostitution involves selling *sex* introduces additional complexities to do with power:

> The buying and selling of sex is not the same as other kinds of transaction if only because we, and the societies we are part of, have such deep-seated and often contradictory notions of sex, and sexuality and its appropriate expression. Furthermore, it is difficult, if not impossible, to separate sex from issues of power and control. These can potentially become highly charged in the context of commercial sex. (p. 106)

Although implicit rather than explicit in this account, these 'issues of power and control' are gendered. That is, they both express and perpetuate gendered relations of power, in a way which is not directly paralleled by care work (although see Lloyd, this volume). The risk to those caring for people with HIV and/or AIDS remains the same regardless of gender[9] but women prostitutes are more vulnerable than their male counterparts to *all* the health risks associated with selling sex, including violence, rape, mental health problems and sexually transmissible diseases (Bloor *et al.*, 1991; Karim *et al.*, 1993; Pyett and Warr, 1996, 1997). For example, although violence from male clients represents a significant occupational health risk for women who sell sex (Barnard and McKeganey, 1996; Pyett and Warr, 1996; Whittaker and Hart, 1996), most male prostitutes are able and willing to defend themselves, and are as likely to present a risk to their clients as vice versa (Bloor *et al.*, 1991). Of particular importance in the context of HIV risk is the relative powerlessness of women sex workers to insist on condom use by their clients (Patton, 1994; Pyett and Warr, 1996).

But perhaps the most poignant consequence of the emotion/commerce distinction is the obligation so clearly felt by women sex workers themselves to mark as clearly as possible the distinction between customers (commerce) and lovers (emotion). Research projects from Australia to South Africa, from Holland to Scotland, reveal very similar patterns of behaviour. Inhabiting the sociocultural boundary zone between emotion and commerce, policed as it is by shame, humiliation, social exclusion, male violence and (usually) the full force of the law, prostitution is a painful and hurtful way to earn a living. Over and over again, women sex workers around the world employ the same potentially dangerous strategy to enable them to protect their sense of privacy and their intimate relationships; they use condoms with paying customers but not with boyfriends, lovers, husbands and partners (Venema and Visser, 1990; Karim et al., 1993; Patton, 1994; Pyett and Warr, 1996, 1997).

Towards a redefinition of occupational health?

The complex social, cultural and sexual-political issues that determine the nature of prostitution and of unpaid care work offer a particularly difficult challenge to occupational health. Both are forms of labour that have traditionally been constructed as non-occupations. There is therefore little recognition of the work-related hazards faced by either group.

Such risks are particularly great for women who sell sex. Decriminalising prositution has demonstrable occupational health benefits for these women. Yet the risks of sex work do not stem solely from its informal and criminalised nature. They have their roots in gendered relations of power, and in a deep-seated anxiety to demarcate the arenas of commerce and affection, and it is this that sex work shares with care work. Herein lies a radical challenge to occupational health. Meeting the occupational health needs of these two groups demands not that health professionals and activists overturn the gendered relations of power or the commerce/affection divide (such tasks are daunting!), but that everyone involved in the field recognises the *constitutive power* that discourses of occupational health inevitably wield, and takes responsibility for this.[10]

In practical terms this means (for example) recognising and challenging the part played by current notions of occupational health in maintaining the emotion/commerce boundary. There are very many problems implicit in regarding selling sex as an ordinary occupation – not the least of which is that to do so risks concealing the power relations expressed in prostitution. There may also be possible dangers in expanding the field of influence of health promotion into the domestic sector; such interventions may (unavoidably?) contain an uncomfortable element of social control (Lupton, 1995).

The transformation required of occupational health, then, does not lie in the direction of professional expansionism. It is not the case that 'occupational health' is a model of proven usefulness which simply requires to be applied to other areas of life. Rather, I have suggested here that it is a discursive construct that acts not only to exclude certain groups of vulnerable workers but also to prop up sociocultural structures such as gender divisions and the commerce/emotion boundary which are themselves counterproductive in terms of health promotion. If this is the case, then what is needed is a critical and radical reflexivity when developing the professional, conceptual and political boundaries of occupational health.

Notes

1   'Universal precautions' is a practice term from health and social care, and refers to the set of precautions that professionals should take *universally*, that is, with every patient/client, in order to prevent transmission of pathogens from patient/client to worker and cross-infection between patients/clients in health and social care settings. They include sterilisation of equipment, precautions for disposal of non-reusable equipment (such as needles and other 'sharps'), use of proper cleaning/disinfecting solutions when mopping up spillages of body fluids, and routine wearing of appropriate protective gear (which may vary, depending on context, from latex or rubber gloves through to plastic aprons, face masks or plastic goggles). Such precautions were supposedly in place as a protection against hepatitis long before HIV became an issue in these settings, although the fears generated about HIV exposed a routine laxity in their use.

2   Although there is a tentative, but developing, 'sociology of the emotions'.

3   Mildred Pearson, mother/carer for a son who died with AIDS, cited in Panos, 1990, p. 60.

4   The buddying system developed among the lesbian and gay communities in the USA and was widely adopted. It involves trained volunteers being assigned to a PWHA to provide practical and emotional support on a regular basis.

5   This must be seen in the context of the professional field of occupational health, which remains fragmented and privatised, and subject to an aggressive rhetoric of deregulation in Britain and elsewhere in Europe. I am grateful to Norma Daykin for making the implications of this situation much clearer to me.

6   This is not to suggest that Euroamerican cultures are alone in scapegoating prostitutes, simply that what follows is an examination of these cultures specifically.

7 This tendency strikes me as being as unhelpful as regarding the virtual slave labour in some third world carpet manufacture as overenthusiastic indulgence in handicrafts. Prostitution bears the same relationship to 'sex' as the exploitation of carpet makers bears to the kind of craft activity enjoyed by many westerners as a hobby.

8 For a discussion of the distinction between decriminalisation and legalisation, see Scrambler and Scrambler, 1995.

9 Unless, that is, there is a sexual relationship between carer and PWHA. However, the significant difference here is that the sexual activity that carries the greatest risk in terms of HIV is getting semen in your anus or vagina (to paraphrase long-time AIDS activist and educator Cindy Patton). It is, therefore, not gender *per se* which is at issue here.

10 To do so may lead to the postmodern ethical position of *responsibility to otherness*, as proposed by White (1991) and elaborated upon by Nick Fox (this volume).

Acknowledgements

Thanks are due to Norma Daykin and Lesley Doyal for their sensitive and rigorous editorial support, and to Priscilla Pyett and Deborah Warr of the Centre for the Study of STDs at La Trobe University in Melbourne for their generosity in sharing their work with me.

References

Abercrombie, N., Warde, A., Soothill, K., Urry, J. and Walby, S. (1994) *Contemporary British Society*, 2nd edn. Cambridge: Polity.
ACTUP New York Women and AIDS Book Group (eds) (1990) *Women, AIDS and Activism*. Boston: South End Press.
Adkins, L. (1995) *Gendered Work: Sexuality, Family and the Labour Market*. Buckingham: Open University Press.
Barnard, M. and McKeganey, N. (1996) 'Prostitution and peer education: beyond HIV' in T. Rhodes and R. Hartnoll (eds), *AIDS, Drugs and Prevention: Perspectives on Individual and Community Action*. London: Routledge.
Berer, M. (with Ray, S.) (eds) (1993) *Women and HIV/AIDS: An International Resource Book*. London: Pandora.
Bloor, M.J., Barnard, M.A., Finlay, A. and McKeganey, N.P. (1991) 'HIV-related risk practices among Glasgow male prostitutes'. Paper presented to the Annual Conference of the British Sociological Association, Manchester.
Boffin, T. and Gupta, S. (eds) (1990) *Ecstatic Antibodies: Resisting the AIDS Mythology*. London: Rivers Oram.
Boseley, S. (1997) 'HIV doctor denies misconduct', *The Guardian*, 11 March, 4.
Brandt, A. (1987) *No Magic Bullet: A Social History of Venereal Disease in the United States since 1880*. Oxford: Oxford University Press.

Centers for Disease Control (1985) *Morbidity and Mortality Weekly Report*, 5 November.

Cockburn, C. (1983) *Brothers: Male Dominance and Technological Change*. London: Pluto.

Cockburn, C. (1985) *Machinery of Dominance: Women, Men and Technical Know-How*. London: Pluto.

Cockburn, C. (1987a) *Women, Trade Unions and Political Parties*. London: Fabian Society.

Cockburn, C. (1987b) *Two-Track Training: Sex Inequalities and the YTS*. London: Macmillan.

DeVita, V.T., Hellman, S. and Rosenberg, S.A. (1988) *AIDS: Etiology, Diagnosis, Treatment and Prevention*. Philadelphia: Lippincott.

Dowling, S. (1994) 'Women have feelings too: the mental health needs of women living with HIV infection' in L. Doyal, J. Naidoo and T. Wilton (eds), *AIDS: Setting a Feminist Agenda*. London: Taylor & Francis.

Doyal, L. (1995) *What Makes Women Sick: Gender and the Political Economy of Health*. London: Macmillan.

Foucault, M. (1979) *Discipline and Punish*. Harmondsworth: Penguin.

Fox, N. (1993) *Postmodernism, Sociology and Health*. Buckingham: Open University Press.

Galbally, R. (ed.) (1997) *VicHealth Letter*, Issue 6, March.

Giddens, A. (1997) *Sociology*, 3rd edn. Cambridge: Polity.

Gilman, S. (1995) *Health and Illness: Images of Difference*. London: Reaktion.

Goss, D. and Adam-Smith, D. (1996) 'HIV/AIDS and employment: a radical critique' *Critical Social Policy*, **16**(48): 77–94.

Graham, H. (1993) *Hardship and Health in Women's Lives*. London: Harvester Wheatsheaf.

Grover, J.Z. (1989) 'Constitutional symptoms' in E. Carter and S. Watney (eds) *Taking Liberties: AIDS and Cultural Politics*. London: Serpent's Tail.

Hobson, B.M. (1987) *Uneasy Virtue: The Politics of Prostitution and the American Reform Tradition*. New York: Basic Books.

Hussey, J. (1996) *Employment and AIDS: A Review of the Companies Act Business Charter on HIV and AIDS*. London: National AIDS Trust.

Karim, Q.A., Karim, S.S.A., Soldan, K. and Zondi, M. (1993) 'Sex work, power and risk of HIV infection'. Unpublished paper, Medical Research Council, South Africa.

Kilpatrick, A. and Kilpatrick, D. (1987) *AIDS*. Edinburgh: Chambers.

Land, H. (1991) 'Time to care' in M. Maclean and D. Groves (eds), *Women's Issues in Social Policy*. London: Routledge.

Leonard, Z. and Thistlethwaite, P. (1990) 'Prostitution and HIV infection' in ACTUP New York Women and AIDS Book Group (eds), *Women, AIDS and Activism*. Boston: South End Press.

Lupton, D. (1995) *The Imperative of Health: Public Health and the Regulated Body*. London: Sage.

Malos, E. (1996) *The Politics of Housework*, 2nd edn. Cheltenham: New Clarion Press.

Manchester AIDSLINE Women's Group (n.d.) *HIV/AIDS and the Under Fives: A Guide for Workers and Carers*. Manchester: Manchester AIDSLINE.

Martin, E. (1987) *The Woman in the Body: A Cultural Analysis of Reproduction*. Buckingham: Open University Press.

Messing, K., Dumais, L. and Romito, P. (1993) 'Prostitutes and chimney sweeps both have problems: towards full integration of both sexes in the study of occupational health', *Social Science and Medicine*, **36**(1): 47–55.

Panos Institute (1990) *Triple Jeopardy: Women and AIDS*. London: Panos.

Pateman, C. (1988) *The Sexual Contract*. Cambridge: Polity.

Patton, C. (1994) *Last Served? Gendering the HIV Pandemic*. London: Taylor & Francis.

Pyett, P. and Warr, D. (1996) 'When "gut instinct" is not enough: women at risk in sex work'. Report to the Community: Melbourne, Centre for the Study of Sexually Transmissible Diseases, La Trobe University.

Pyett, P. and Warr, D. (1997) 'Vulnerability on the streets: female sex workers and HIV risk', *AIDS Care*.

Richardson, D. (1989) *Women and the AIDS Crisis*, 2nd edn. London: Pandora.

Scambler, G. and Scambler, A. (1995) 'Social change and health promotion among women sex workers in London', *Health Promotion International*, **10**(1): 17–24.

Terry, J. and Urla, J. (eds) (1995) *Deviant Bodies: Critical Perspectives on Difference in Science and Popular Culture*. Bloomington: Indiana University Press.

Treichler, P. (1988) 'AIDS, gender and biomedical discourse: current contests for meaning' in E. Fee and D. Fox (eds), *AIDS: The Burdens of History*. Berkeley: University of California Press.

Turner, B. (1995) *Medical Power and Social Knowledge*. London: Sage.

Venema, P.U. and Visser, J. (1990) 'Safer prostitution: a new approach in Holland' in M. Plant (ed.) *AIDS, Drugs and Prostitution*. London: Routledge.

Waldby, C. (1996) *AIDS and the Body Politic: Biomedicine and Sexual Difference*. London: Routledge.

Wells, J. (1982) *A Herstory of Prostitution in Western Europe*. Berkeley: Shameless Hussy Press.

White, S. (1991) *Political Theory and Postmodernism*. Cambridge: Cambridge University Press.

Whittaker, D. and Hart, G. (1996) 'Research note: managing risks: the social organisation of indoor sex work', *Sociology of Health and Illness*, **18**(3): 399–414.

Wilson, J. (1993) 'Women as carers, Scotland' in M. Berer (with S. Ray) (eds), *Women and HIV/AIDS: An International Resource Book*. London: Pandora.

Wilton, T. (1992) *Antibody Politic: AIDS and Society*. Cheltenham: New Clarion.

Wilton, T. (1997) *En/Gendering AIDS: Deconstructing Sex, Texts, Epidemic*. London: Sage.

11 POSTMODERN REFLECTIONS: DECONSTRUCTING 'RISK', 'HEALTH' AND 'WORK'

Nick J. Fox

Following on from the previous analysis of risk discourses, this chapter presents the case for a radical rethinking of notions of risk. The limitations of the realist position, in which risks are presumed to be knowable and controllable through the application of scientific methods and rigorous management, are explored. The objectivity of this approach is revealed to be illusory, and the power relationships and moral classifications which underlie it are examined from a post-modern perspective. Exploring this perspective in more depth, the author emphasises the possibility of choice and resistance to discourses as individuals' own lives and agendas unfold.

Risk, modernity and reflexivity

Risk, in the sense in which it is now understood, is a peculiarly modern concept. Before the period of modernity (which can be said to have begun around about 1800), *risk* was a neutral term, concerned merely with probabilities, of losses and gains. A gamble or an endeavour which was associated with high risk meant simply that there was great potential for significant loss or significant reward. However, in the modern period, *risk* has been coopted as a term reserved for the negative outcome alone, and has supplanted the terms *danger* or *hazard*. Thus the British Medical Association's (1987) guide *Living with Risk* describes a *hazard* as 'a set of circumstances which may cause harmful consequences', while *risk* is 'the likelihood of its doing so' (p. 13). Furthermore, this hazard/risk differentiation introduces a moral dimension, such that the perpetrators of *risk* may be held to account in some way or other (Douglas, 1992, pp. 22–5).

Such accounting, so typical of the Weberian rationalisations of modernism (Fox, 1991; Prior, 1995, p. 134), provides the basis for a new science of risk calculation, from the actuarial tables of life insurers, to the risk analysis of those in the (literal) business of risk: the movers and shakers of capitalism. In what might almost be a handbook for such entrepreneurial activity, Johnstone-Bryden (1995), in a monograph sub-titled *How to Work Successfully with Risk* offers a blueprint for 'how risks can be identified and reduced economically and effectively, before serious damage occurs' (p. 1).

Risk assessment, we are led to believe by such authors, is a technical procedure which like all aspects of modern life is to be undertaken through rational calculation of ends and means (Fox, 1991). Figure 11.1 is taken from a UK government publication on risk assessment (Department of the Environment, 1995). It shows the 'simple, logical sequence of steps' (p. 5) to be taken to identify and manage risk. This process of risk assessment has been widely applied to many areas of technology over the past half century (Carter, 1995, p. 135). Within such a scenario, all risks may be evaluated and suitably managed, such that all may be predicted and countered, so risks, accidents and insecurities are minimised or prevented altogether (Johnstone-Bryden, 1995, p. 3; Prior, 1995).

However, such accounts ignore the socially constructed and historically specific character of such conceptualisations. At the simplest level, we may conclude that 'risk is in the eye of the beholder'

> Insurance experts (involuntarily) contradict safety engineers. While the latter diagnose zero risk, the former decide: uninsurable. Experts are undercut or deposed by opposing experts. Politicians encounter the resistance of citizens' groups, and industrial management encounters morally and politically motivated organized consumer boycotts. (Beck, 1994, p. 11)

Ulrich Beck has called the period we now inhabit in the west the era of 'reflexive modernization', and has typified it as a 'risk society' (Beck, 1992, 1994). In a risk society, the proliferation of risks as a consequence of the rapidity of society's technological innovation has got out of control. The success of modernist instrumental rationality has led to an apparent solution through technology to every problem, ill or need.

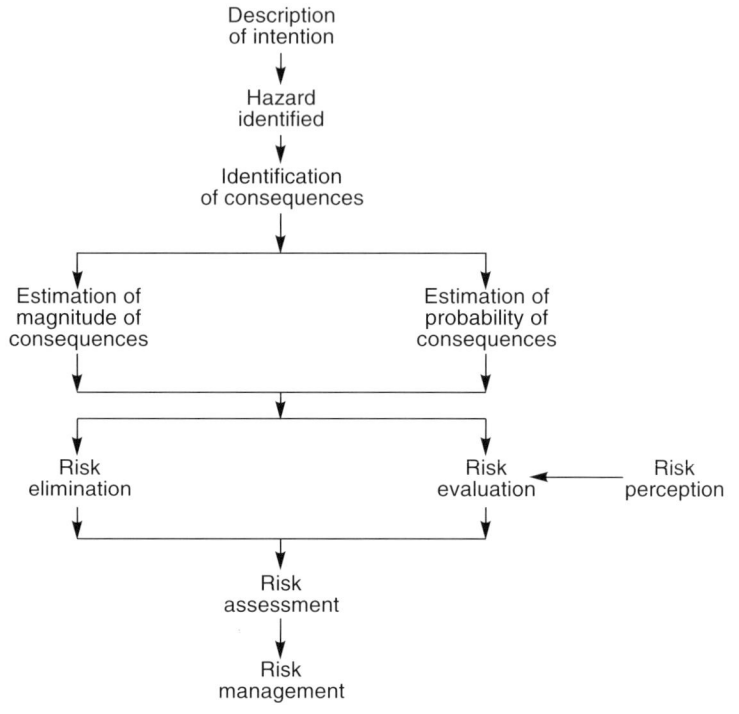

Figure 11.1   From intention to risk management

Source: Department of the Environment, 1995

But alongside the development of technology, and – for those who make a living through such innovation – the accumulation of wealth, Beck suggests there is a concomitant accumulation of risks in undesirable abundance: radioactivity, toxins and pollutants, all kinds of hazards associated with working with or consuming technology (1992, pp. 22, 26). But, Beck goes on, risks:

> only exist in terms of the (scientific or anti-scientific) knowledge about them. They can be changed, magnified, dramatized or minimized within knowledge, and to that extent they are particularly open to social definition and construction. (Beck, 1992, p. 23, original emphases)

Furthermore, some people are more affected by the distribution and growth of risks, and there are winners and losers in risk definitions.

Power and access to and control of knowledge thus become paramount in a risk society. This is the issue of *reflexivity* to which Beck alludes: society becomes a problem for itself (Beck, 1994, p. 8). Further:

> In risk issues, no one is an expert, or everyone is an expert, because all the experts presume what they are supposed to make possible and produce: cultural acceptance. The Germans see the world perishing along with their forests. The Britons are shocked by their toxic breakfast eggs: this is where and how their ecological conversion starts. (p. 9)

This, for Beck, is both a crisis for society in the late modern period, and an opportunity for social critique, and ultimately for a new emancipation coming in the wake of the failure of socialism to provide a resolution to the inequities of capitalism (Beck, 1994, p. 12). Reflexivity challenges the old status barriers of class and control of wealth, creating new possibilities for coalition and organisation.

This kind of analysis is based in realism or 'scientism', and does not really address the impact of culture on the construction of risk as a concept (Lash, 1994, pp. 199–200). For Beck, the focus on reflexivity is at the level of the organisation, not upon the sense-making activities of subjects. Along with other social theorists working in the *poststructuralist* or *postmodern* tradition, I am more interested in the effects of a reflexive society upon individuals and their subjectivities. In the chapter, I explore this aspect of the social construction of risk, asking some questions about the fabrication of 'risk' as a concept, in relation to the other topics relevant to this book: 'health' and 'work'.

At the 'cultural' end of the spectrum of social theories of risk, Mary Douglas's work has been highly influential. In a recent paper (Douglas, 1992), she offers an historical account of how an anthropologist such as herself came to be interested in risk, which supplies a further angle on the reflexivity of late modernism. She describes her surprise in the 1970s when a 'modern' society seemed to respond to fears over pollution in much the same way as the 'tribes' she had studied for her *Purity and Danger* and other writing on taboos (Douglas, 1966). Despite the proliferation of risk research and the founding of an academic discipline for communicating risks:

> The baffling behaviour of the public, in refusing to buy floodplain or earthquake insurance, in crossing dangerous roads, driving non-road-worthy vehicles, buying accident-provoking gadgets for the home, and not listening to the education on risks, all that continues as before. (Douglas, 1992, p. 11)

Douglas suggested that the reason such behaviour seems baffling is the failure to take culture into account. She sought to illustrate how the risks one focused upon as an individual had less to do with individual psychology (the discipline informing rational choice theory and the health belief model) and more about the social forms in which those individuals construct their understanding of the world and themselves (Douglas, 1992, p. 12). Further:

> If the cultural processes by which certain societies select certain kinds of dangers for attention are based on institutional procedures for allocating responsibility, for self-justification, or for calling others to account, it follows that public moral judgments will advertise certain risks powerfully, while the well-advertised risk will turn out to be connected with legitimating moral principles. (Rayner, 1992, p. 92)

In her earlier work Douglas (1973) developed a typology of cultures based on the two dimensions of *grid* and *group* (reflecting degrees of social stratification and social solidarity respectively). Three of the four possible combinations of high and low grid and group are identified by Douglas in her most recent work (and developed and explored in Rayner, 1992) as cultural backcloths to risk decisions and perceptions (the fourth – high grid/low group – comprises isolated, alienated individuals). Douglas suggests that they are all reflected in (late) modern culture, and her typology (with some adaptations of mine) is illustrated in Table 11.1. The low grid/low group culture is typical of the competitive environment of the entrepreneurial capitalist free market, in which individuals are untrammelled by restrictive practices or rules. Also found in capitalist institutions are the high grid/high group cultures where Weber's 'iron cage' of bureaucracy has regulated and incorporated systems and structures for interaction. The third kind of culture, low grid/high group are collectivistic, egalitarian groups, which Douglas and others have suggested are found in voluntary groups including the anti-nuclear movement and political and religious cults (Douglas, 1992, p. 77; Rayner, 1992, p. 89).

With these different cultures in mind, what is considered as a risk, and how great that risk is seen to be, will be dependent upon the organisation or grouping to which a person belongs or identifies, as will the perceived causes of disasters, accidents or other negative occurrences which occur. Where reflection turns inward upon the organisation itself, blame will be ascribed in different ways and to different targets. This typology has been developed and related to empirical examples. Thus, for example, Douglas (1992, pp. 102–21) explores the impact of these cultural dimensions of stratification and solidarity upon indi-

Table 11.1 A typology of cultures of risk perception

	Market (low grid/low group)	Bureaucratic (high grid/high group)	Voluntary (low grid/high group)
Latent goal	Individual freedom to contract	Internal structure of authority	Survival of group
Organisational objective in interpreting disasters	Enhance competitiveness	Enhance control over individuals	Dampen dissidence or clarify factions
Risks perceived in terms of	Competitors' innovations or business advantage	Punitive outside environment	External betrayals/conspiracies
Internal enquiries blame	Failure in leadership or team members	Loss of group commitment	Individual treachery

Source: Adapted from Douglas, 1992

vidual health responses to HIV contagion. The emphasis in this culturalist model of risk perception upon the *social* construction of risk is
highly relevant for the explorations which follow.

Health at work: three models of the risk/hazard opposition

At the beginning of this chapter, I remarked upon the constructions of
risk and *hazard* in modernist discourse. Having explored the different
positions of realist and culturalist analysts (as exemplified by Beck and
Douglas), I now want to look at this in somewhat greater depth in relation to issues of health at work, to consider the differing perspectives
which are possible concerning the ontological relation of a *risk* to a
hazard. I shall consider three possibilities, the last of which being what
I shall call the *postmodern* position, with its emphasis on the textual
fabrication of reality.

Position 1: The risk maps directly on to the underlying hazard

The first position might be called realist or materialist, given the underlying ontology of a hazard as real and material, and is the perspective
identified at the beginning of the chapter, as the mapping of a *risk* (that
is, the likelihood of an unpleasant occurrence) upon a *hazard*, (the
circumstances which could lead to the occurrence). Thus the risks for
health workers of contracting hepatitis or other blood-related diseases
are directly linked to (among other things) the hazard of working with
sharps (hypodermic needles and so on). Given the existence of sharps
in the work environment of a hospital nurse or doctor, then there will
be a probability of an accidental needlestick injury, and given that a
proportion of patients will be positive for a blood-transmitted disease,
there will be a probability that in the event of an accident, a health
worker will be infected.

 This is the position which is generally adopted in risk management
and assessment literature, where the objective is risk reduction. Given
the presence of the hazard in the work environment, then strategies
are to be adopted to minimise the likelihood (the risk) that the hazard
will be manifested in an unpleasant outcome. The emphasis may be on
individual education, individual or population prevention measures or
corporate strategy. As such, the position is not inherently political, and
may be coopted to serve any or all of the different interests which may
engage discursively with the perceived hazard.

Rogers and Salvage (1988) reproduce a Royal College of Nursing poster concerning contamination:

HEPATITIS B IS A NEEDLEsS RISK

Take our advice. Get vaccinated

This emphasises personal responsibility for risk reduction in the face of a hazard. The authors follow this up with a list of hazards, commenting that:

> Staff working in higher risk areas are usually (though not always) aware of the hazards, and should be well versed in procedures for dealing with them... Nurses must therefore be aware which patients could be carriers of the virus. They include... (Rogers and Salvage, 1988, p. 103)

From a campaigning position, the London Hazards Centre writes, concerning its publication of a handbook raising issues concerning computer screens (VDUs) that:

> The headaches, eye strain, vision problems, stress and musculo-skeletal disorders suffered by VDU workers were caused by a combination of badly-designed jobs, equipment and working environments, and that most of the conditions could be prevented by rigorous attention to the way in which jobs were organised, and by the provision of appropriate equipment and workplaces. (London Hazards Centre, 1993, p. 1)

And, from a corporate perspective, Johnstone-Bryden suggests that:

> People represent the real risk. Human greed, malice and error are the primary threats. It could be argued that almost every risk, perhaps even every risk, relates back to human error, or deliberate human actions. (Johnstone-Bryden, 1995, p. 57)

While the realist or materialist position may acknowledge that the level of risk offered by a hazard is based on subjective judgement, the one-to-one mapping of risk on to hazard means that, while:

> At no time will all of us agree on a single level of acceptable risk... if people can agree upon the way risks are measured, and on the relevance of the levels of risk thus represented to the choices we must all make, then the scope for disagreement and dissent is thereby limited. (British Medical Association, 1987, p. vii)

Despite the different value perspectives of analysts (for example, from management, trade unions or pressure groups), the realist position establishes the potential for a formal process of scientific analysis of risks. I would suggest that such a claimed consensus over *how* to assess risk also creates the basis for moral judgements concerning implementation of risk reduction procedures, and implicitly, a culture of blame (although, as Douglas' typology implies, who is blamed may depend on who the analyst is).

Position 2: Hazards are natural, risks are cultural

In the second position, which might be called culturalist or constructionist, risks are opposed to hazards in the sense that while the latter are 'natural' and neutral, risks are the value-laden judgements of human beings concerning these natural events or possibilities. Within social science, this approach to risk has become more prominent, and if we may once again focus on Mary Douglas, despite her culturalist analysis which seeks to demonstrate that risks are perceived in a social context, she is keen to note that:

> The dangers are only too horribly real... this argument is not about the reality of the dangers, but about how they are politicized ...Starvation, blight and famine are perennial threats. It is a bad joke to take this analysis as hinting that the dangers are imaginary. (Douglas, 1992, p. 29)

This position has been the basis for a corpus of sociological analyses of risk perception, including many related to health and illness (for instance the recent collections by Gabe, 1995 and Bunton *et al.*, 1995). Two main themes emerge: one concerning the differing types of 'knowledge' which inform perceptions of risk, and the second the moral dimension to risk and risk taking.

Looking once again at the issue of exposure to infectious diseases by health workers, and taking some material from my own study of surgery (Fox, 1992), the dangers of infection by hepatitis or HIV were problematic for health workers in operating theatres, because by their nature, the hazards were invisible and unquantifiable. Rarely were patients known to be positive for a hazardous blood-communicated disease, and trust was therefore crucial within the hospital work environment for establishing risk perceptions. An operating department manager said:

> It's always possible that a patient with HIV or hepatitis will come in. Staff need to be convinced that the precautions are as foolproof as we can make them, but there is always a risk. (Nurse Manager F)

The degree of professional commitment seemed to affect the trust which staff might have in the workplace, so that:

> With the orderlies and junior nursing staff there is a need for psychological counselling to cope with the risk. (Nurse Manager F)

Anaesthetist Dr J suggested that the issue of possible contamination was silently acknowledged by medical staff, and the use of protective eye guards by a surgeon might implicitly indicate that a patient was high risk, and additional precautions should be taken by all involved in the procedure. (This comment was made during an operation in which a tattoo was removed from a young woman's arm – the implication being that such an individual could be positive for hepatitis or HIV.)

Thorogood (1995) noted similar reflections on trust in a survey of patients' reflections on an imagined scenario of attending an HIV-positive dentist. She found patients keen to rely upon the professionalism of the dentist, not only to tell them if they were positive for the disease, but also because it was the dentist who possessed the professional knowledge of the risks involved. In return, they judged themselves responsible for reporting to their dentist if they – the patients – were HIV positive.

In another study of health workers and contamination by blood, Grinyer (1995) explored differences between 'expert' and 'lay' discourses on the prevention of accidental contact with blood products. While the hospital authorities issued advice to staff, in many instances, needlestick accidents had occurred. Staff were doubtful about how feasible it would be to avoid hazards, while some were cynical about the management's need to turn a profit. Grinyer found when she reported some accidents involving sharps and blood products, management denied her data's validity (1995, p. 40). She concluded that such unwillingness to recognise lay knowledge about hazards undermines risk reduction policies. The naiveté of risk assessors must be substituted with a sophisticated sociological account, because:

> Not only are risk perceptions multi-dimensional, but, at any given time, people are managing a number of different agendas which may conflict with the official ones and can be contradictory. Official information is only one of a number of different routes through which a hazard is understood. Powerful social forces shape the way in which information is perceived and acted upon... which may be underestimated by those responsible for risk assessment. (Grinyer, 1995, p. 49)

Grinyer invokes Brian Wynne's analysis of expert knowledge to analyse these discrepancies, arguing that 'expertise' is often held by the lay actors, while expert knowledge is usually based only upon 'scientific evidence'. The 'real world' of a hazard may in this sense be distanced from the naive formal analysis of it in expert discourse (Wynne, 1992, p. 285). I will return to this point in the next section.

The second kind of conclusion reached by the culturalist position concerns the moral character of the risky individual. When Thorogood (1995) reports her respondents making such remarks as 'he wears gloves, uses a mask and a sterilising unit, all you would expect from a good dentist' or 'he is a particularly nice dentist, everything is covered up', the moral implications are clear: the moral qualities of the dentist are indicative of her/his hazardousness. Rogers and Salvage (1988, p. 106) report the other side of the coin, when they describe the stigmatising by her manager of a nurse who had received a needlestick injury, and was required to use a marked cup, saucer and plate, even prior to a test result for HIV. While this is an extreme case, the responsibilities of employees to work 'safely' are at the heart of Health and Safety legislation, and failure to abide by such regulations may lead to victim-blaming. As Simon Carter argues:

> Those groups facing danger which can be defined as 'other' often face controls which work in the interests of the powerful 'same'. Thus a range of social practices exist, connected with risk assessment, which historically have often targeted specific groups... the effect is to push the group into a space of danger – the place of the 'other'. Here they become a useful repository for our cultural ideas of danger. As long as we are 'good'... then danger is elsewhere. (Carter, 1995, pp. 142–3)

A second aspect to the moral dimension of risk concerns the allocation of resources within society to reduce the risks of various hazards. Risk reduction is a cost to industry like any other, and judgements must be made about the relative balance between profitability and safety. Both Wynne's commentary on the undervaluing of non-scientific 'expertise', and the typology developed by Douglas which we examined earlier have significance here, as different agencies will place differing weightings into this equation, depending upon their perspectives. From the culturalist perspective, what is required is a sociologically informed risk assessment, which can overcome the 'naiveté' of the technical scientific evaluation, and take into account the 'real world' of hazards, and how they impinge on the daily working lives of employees.

Position 3: Risk perceptions fabricate hazards

The third position is the one which I shall call postmodern. It moves beyond the culturalist or constructionist model, to argue radically that hazards are *themselves* social fabrications, the reifications of moral judgements about the 'riskiness' of choices made by human beings. These 'hazards' are then invoked discursively to support these estimations of risk and of the people who are associated with them.

To give an example of what may – at first sight – appear counterfactual, let me once again consider the issue of health workers and infected sharps. Let us accept that discarded needles and other sharps which may have been infected by blood products exist as real objects (although this assumption is not of great relevance). In and of themselves, they do not constitute a hazard. However, they become *hazardous* under certain circumstances, principally if conditions arise such that they may come into contact with and pierce the skin of a person in their vicinity. However, the transformation of this 'inert' object into a *hazard* occurs as a consequence of a particular discourse: that of risk assessment (or equivalent lay evaluation of danger or security). It is only in the analysis of risks, that the *hazard* comes into existence: were the risk assessment to be zero or close to zero, the inert object would remain just that.

There are some important consequences from this analysis. First, if we look back at Figure 11.1, which was the flow diagram offered in a Department of the Environment publication, it becomes clear that this explanation of the process of risk assessment and management is inadequate. The selection of various 'inert' objects, procedures or humans as 'hazards' must depend upon some prior judgement, otherwise risk assessors would be faced with an insurmountable task of sifting through every element of an environment or context. Risk analysts in a workplace would be for ever suggesting 'Yes, well, it is feasible that a paperclip could, if accidentally heated to incandescence by sunlight magnified through a skylight, cause a very serious facial scar to anyone deciding to take a nap on their office desk and etc., etc.' Inevitably, risk assessment must begin with some prior knowledge about the world, what is 'probable' and what 'unlikely', what is 'serious', what is 'trivial'. Such judgements may derive from 'scientific' sources, or may depend on common sense or experiential resources. Whatever the source, the judgements will be evaluative, and will derive from the particular knowledgeability utilised by the risk analyst, whether 'expert' or lay.

From this it may be concluded that the objectivity of risk assessment is illusory, and at best is based on some sort of consensus model of the world. However, I noted in the previous section that certain know-ledgeabilities tend to be privileged in the discursive activity of risk assessment. At this point I want to return to Wynne's commentary concerning the world view of risk assessors, which he describes as based upon a naive model of the social world (1992, p. 285). Discussing a risk assessment of pesticide manufacture, Wynne argues that:

> Scientific risk analysis did not avoid, and could not have avoided, making social assumptions in order to create the necessary scientific knowledge. It was *conditional* knowledge in that its validity depended, *inter alia* upon the conditions in this embedded social model being fulfilled in actual practice... Each party, both scientists and workers, tacitly defined different actual risk systems. They built upon different models of the social practices controlling the contaminants and exposures. (Wynne, 1992, pp. 285–6)

Wynne's argument is that scientific, technical discourses tend to make claims to objectivity based on non-real world scenarios, while they tell the public how 'stupid and irrational they are' (p. 286). But this is based not on experts' arrogance, but in a failure to recognise the contingency of their discourse. Such an analysis explains the failure of different groups to agree on risks: not because they have different data, but because they have different knowledgeabilities such that they cannot even agree on what is a hazard. We are led back to Douglas's typology, but now we see that it is not outlooks on *risks* which are dependent on social milieu, but world views on *hazards* (that is, the discursively constructed objects, processes or humans in the environment) themselves. *Both risks and hazards are cultural products.*

A second consequence of the discursive construction of *hazards* follows from this, and is of great significance in addressing issues of 'health' at 'work'. If hazards are constructed not from some real material attributes of the world, but from contingent and partial descriptions of the world as outlined in one or other system of knowledgeability, then the consequent attribution of riskiness is grounded not in objective estimation, but entirely upon what Foucault (1980) calls *power-knowledge*, the knowledgeability which both discursively constructs objects and confirms the authority of the person claiming the knowledge. And, as Foucault has illustrated in his analyses of modern power, it is not only inanimate objects which are constructed in this discursive activity, but also subjectivities.

This needs a few words of explanation. Systems of knowledge are often – tangentially or centrally – about people, how they think about themselves and how they see themselves in relation to the world and to other people. Thus medical knowledge constructs people as patients, the law constructs people as 'criminals' or 'law-abiding subjects', Christianity constructs people as 'sinners'. Modernity, with its emphasis on rationality and scientific knowledge, has created us all as subjects of a myriad systems of knowledge which impinge upon the most intimate aspects of life, including our personal relationships (Foucault, 1970, 1981). Our sense of who we are and how we should behave is the result of countless discourses, both in scientific journals and in popular magazines and the media.

Relating this back to issues of risk, discourses of 'health promotion' have been criticised for suggesting that virtually any action or practice may possess inherent risks to health or wellbeing. Sociological studies have identified the consequent construction of a range of negative subjectivities: the general evaluation as a 'risk taker' or 'risky' individual; 'back slider', in relation to safer sex practices; and the double-edged 'fitness fanatic' (see for example Glassner, 1989; Scott and Freeman, 1995). Demonstrating the capacity to look after one's own body within a discourse on 'lifestyle' has become not only an indicator of self-control, but an important marker of moral worth (Petersen, 1994). Jane Ogden (1995) calls this emphasis upon self-care a move towards an 'intra-active' identity, compartmentalized into a controlling self and a risky self:

> The risk to health comes from the individual's presence or absence of self-control which manages and masters the changeable drives that expose the body to threats. The HIV virus is no longer a risk to health: the individual's ability to control their sexual behaviour is now the risk... In the late twentieth century, the individual has become at risk from his or herself. (Ogden, 1995, p. 413)

While not all risk assessment is oriented towards personal risks, health risks associated with work – as in health promotion – are, by definition, risks to people. Risk assessment establishes the subjectivity of those it addresses as individuals or populations 'at risk'. This is clear as soon as one looks at safety at work literature. Regardless of whether the intention of an author is to set out regulations, advise on safe practice, or alert workers to dangers in their workplace which managers have ignored or downplayed, the work environment is discovered to be a vast repository of risks. Making the connection with Ogden's analysis, workers are 'at risk' on many fronts, and to the extent to which these risks are related to work *practices*, they are 'at risk from themselves', reliant upon the balance between the 'controlling self' and the 'risky self'.

Unlike the previous analyses, in which hazards are assumed to be the 'natural' underpinning of the cultural attribution of risk, in this postmodern position, discourses on the 'hazardous' quality of the environment become possible only through the contingent knowledgeabilities which variously construct a subjectivity in workers as 'at risk'. In the final section of this chapter, I want to explore the impact of this construction of subjectivity, and how it might be possible to refuse and resist it.

'Health' at 'work': choices and refusals

Were health an absolute, then the creation of a subjectivity which would tend to encourage healthy living could be accepted as a necessary evil. Indeed, the modernist discourses of biomedicine and its allies in the social sciences have sought to claim just such an absolutism for 'health' (Fox, 1993). However, just as 'risks' and 'hazards' turn out to be socially constructed in discourses of this or that group, so it is with health.

Health is now rarely defined simply as an absence of illness. The World Health Organisation (WHO, 1985) speaks of health as a state of 'complete physical, mental and social well-being', while Wright (1982) suggests an anthropological phenomenology of 'what it is to function as a human' with illness – somewhat paradoxically – defined as circumstances of a failure to function which continues to be seen as human. Canguilhem (1989) sees health and illness as positive and negative biological values, and Kelly and Charlton call it a 'neutral idea relating to non-pathological physical functioning and the fulfilment of ordinary social roles' (Kelly and Charlton, 1995, p. 83). Illness is a 'notion of increasing dependency' for de Swaan (1990, p. 220), and Sedgewick identified illnesses as socially constructed definitions of natural circumstances which precipitate death or a failure to function within certain norms (1982, p. 30).

We saw earlier the moral dimension to attributions of 'risk', which are generally seen as the negative pole of an opposition to a desired state of 'safety'. Such moral positions are political, in that they ascribe rights and responsibilities to those subjected to them, and require actions commensurate with these rights or responsibilities. The human subject of risk analysis is drawn into a *subjectivity* as 'risky' and perhaps culpable. Similarly, all these definitions of health (be they medical or sociological) have a politics associated with them, all try to persuade us to adopt a particular perspective on the person who is healthy or ill. (All could be deconstructed, had I the space.) Such discourses contribute to the modernist enterprise of mastery: once defined, it is possible to control and change a phenomenon (typically, in this case, from 'ill' to 'healthy'). This modernist responsibility to act replaces any concern with the justice of the action in and of itself (Bauman, 1989). This responsibility, Stephen White suggests:

> Always requires one, at some point, to fix or close down parameters of thought or ignore or homogenize at least some dimensions of specificity or difference among actors. (White, 1991, p. 21)

White goes on to argue that the postmodern politic is the substitution of this responsibility to act with a *responsibility to otherness*. The need for such an ethos concerning health and care is highlighted in the work of Oliver Sacks, who has documented the refusals and rejections of medicalising definitions of health and illness among his patients. An artist who lost his colour sight refused a chance to restore it, having developed a way of seeing and creating in monochrome (Sacks, 1995). A person with Tourette's Syndrome found that his medication not only removed his erratic behaviour but destroyed much of what he valued in himself as a person (Sacks, 1985). The 'awakening' of people treated with L-Dopa for their Parkinsonism was, in some cases, a horrifying experience as they were confronted with 'reality' (Sacks, 1991). We must ask how many people are persuaded into 'cures' which cut across their subjectivity, inscribing a new medical identity – with no acknowledgement of their 'right' to otherness.

So a responsibility to otherness, in relation to issues of 'health' and 'illness', will suggests a radically different conception of human potential, and I have coined the term *arche-health* (Fox, 1993) to denote this. *Arche-health* is a 'becoming' rather than a being, a process not a state, a resistance to discourse and a subjectivity untrammelled by obligation to be something or other. It is not intended to suggest a natural, essential or in any way prior kind of health, upon which the other healths are superimposed, it is not supposed to be a rival concept, indeed the reason for using this rather strange term is its homage to Derrida's (1976, p. 56) notion of *arche-writing*, which is not writing but that which supplied the possibility of writing, that is, the system of difference upon which language is based. Similarly, *arche-health*:

- is the becoming of the organism which made it possible for the first time to speak of health or illness
- is present, in the sense that a trace of it is carried, in every discourse on health
- can never become the object of scientific investigation, without falling back into discourse on health/illness
- is multiple in its effects. As difference, it is meaningless to speak of its unity or its division
- reminds us to ask hard questions of the modernist disciplines which inscribe us through their conceptions of, and preoccupations with, 'health' and 'illness'.

There is not room here to explore the wider issues of *arche-health*, how one can move towards it, and how to refuse the discourses of 'health (for further reading, see Fox, 1993, 1995, 1997a). But the reason for introducing it here in relation to health at work follows from the earlier discussions of how discourses of risk construct subjectivities in those who are implicated – in the context of this chapter – people at work.

It has become unfashionable in sociology to speak of choices. Both Marxist and Weberian traditions emphasised the constraints on action, and the Foucauldian discourse on the construction of the self has described a human subject seemingly incapable of resistance (Lash, 1991; Fox, 1997b). Postmodern approaches (including those engaging with feminism) have sought to reintroduce discussions of how it is possible to refuse the totalizing effects of discourse (Deleuze and Guattari, 1984, 1988; Butler, 1990; Cixous, 1990), and the notion of *arche-health* as a resistance, a *becoming-other*, articulates with these writings. Choice, however, appears so relevant in relation to work and health, perhaps precisely because work seems like an area of life which is so often done unwillingly, as a necessity in a capitalist, oppressive (in a Marxist sense) society (BMA, 1987, p. 67). There is thus a sense in which it is particularly 'unfair' or immoral if, as a consequence of working, one's health is affected, because 'health' is claimed as a basic human right (Kelly and Charlton, 1995, p. 83). Indeed, within a narrow sense of 'health' as variously defined earlier, I would of course, agree with such an evaluation.

But if we acknowledge the constructed nature of these 'healths', (and you could deconstruct the moral and political bases for any of the notions of health and illness documented earlier), we see how the subjectivity which arises from each is based in a partial truth grounded in some claim or other concerning what it is to be a human being, or have a body, or be part of a community, or whatever. This is where choice comes in, although not in an individualistic, rational-actor sense. Rather, choice may be exerted negatively, in a refusal or resistance, as well as positively in affirmations. Choices may be temperamental or unconscious, or collective, as opposed to rational or individual. But such choosings are processual, and are associated with the arche-health I spoke of before, in that they are a becoming rather than a state of being.

Let me illustrate the point I wish to make with regard to health at work with an example from my study of surgical work, and the hazards of blood-transmitted infection:

> Surgeon Mr T: Never a month goes by that we don't nick ourselves with a scalpel or other instrument, and I suppose we should be concerned about the risk, but we don't generally do anything.
>
> Researcher: I suppose the gloves offer some protection?
>
> Mr T: Yes, once a week I tear a glove, so they may help.
>
> Researcher: Do you take precautions when you have a patient who might be a risk?
>
> Mr T: Well, it's only if there is inoculation of blood that it's a problem.
>
> Researcher: What about blood spray into the eyes?
>
> Mr T: That can be a danger, I suppose. I often wear lenses (binocular magnifiers) so they have a double use. (Fox, 1992, p. 29)

Mr T, as with other other surgeons studied, seems blasé about hazards which are present in his work environment. He could take various actions to reduce these if he wished but all have costs associated with them, and ultimately he makes choices to continue to do a job which he wishes to do, trying to reduce the likelihood of infection where he perceives a higher risk. Work for Mr T is not simply something which he is coerced into, it is the result of a series of choices which he, and his associates, make on a daily basis. Recall too the earlier extracts concerning 'professionalism' and infection, which suggest the choices made by grades of nursing staff based on different perspectives on their work and their responsibilities to others. Mr T is *active* in his living out of a set of activities which are called 'work' and which impinge upon certain facets of the continuity of that life called 'health'. He makes positive and negative choices concerning how he acts and how we sees himself in relation to his work setting and his associates and patients. His evaluations of hazards are based in these complex choices and perceptions, and are part of his *becoming-other* and his *arche-health* as he lives. We need to recognise that 'work' too is a socially constructed category, and can be constituted variously: for instance to include or exclude voluntary activities, professional sport and educational studies. Work can only be defined contingently, within discourses which establish certain ethical and political regimes of 'truth', within particular knowledgeabilities, and with particular objectives.

Conclusions: threats and opportunities

Risk, health and work are all concepts which form part of a set of discourses on modern life. They are tied up with the values of a culture and the moral rights and responsibilities of members of that same culture, and as such are implicated in how people understand themselves as reflective, ethical subjects. Such a postmodern reflection is intrinsically political, addressing the power relations of a society which may be, as Beck (1992) suggests, productive of 'risk'. Its politics are radical in that – in deconstructing these relations – it offers a means to resist them.

We have seen how risks are not absolutes, neither are the 'hazards' which are supposedly the circumstances which constitute risks. Both are tied up with the valorisations of certain kinds of living, and the ideas of health and work which are constructed in a 'risk society' are at the same time dependent upon ideas of risk and constitutive of 'risk' itself. We implicitly evaluate certain actions or situations in terms of the consequences for ourselves or others and label these actions or situations as more or less threatening to our physical, psychological or moral integrity. Similarly we weigh these up in making assessments of work, with – paradoxically – hazardous jobs either highly or very poorly paid (for mortality rates in different occupations see *BMA*, 1987, p. 68).

What I have sought to show is that because these conceptions are contingent, the subjectivities which are created around risk, health and work are relative, and grounded in discursive fabrications of what is to be positively or negatively valued. I believe it offers an additional perspective to the realist and culturalist positions described in the chapter. It focuses on the social processes involved in risk assessment, but addresses the impact on the individual, and offers a perspective on risk as the active process of choosing as life unfolds: a *becoming-other* and a resistance to discourse. The implication is that it is neither sufficient to point to phenomena and claim they are hazardous (because such claims are always dependent on the world view of the claimant), nor to assume that by making such claims one is necessarily acting in the interests of those whom one may be trying to assist.

As a perspective, the postmodern view is not intended to challenge the critiques of industrial production as often injurious to the bodies, minds and spirits of individuals, but to suggest that the becoming of body, mind or spirit needs to be seen as processual. Health and work are constituted in the unfolding lives of individuals with their own agendas: differently formulated, a risk can – in the right circumstances – be an opportunity to become other.

References

Bauman, Z. (1989) Modernity and the Holocaust. Cambridge: Polity.

Beck, U. (1992) *Risk Society*. London: Sage.

Beck, U. (1994) 'The reinvention of politics: towards a theory of reflexive modernization' in U. Beck, A. Giddens, and S. Lash (eds), *Reflexive Modernization*. Cambridge: Polity.

British Medical Association (1987) *Living with Risk*. Chichester: John Wiley.

Bunton, R., Nettleton, S. and Burrows, R. (eds) (1995) *The Sociology of Health Promotion*. London: Routledge

Butler, J. (1990) *Gender Trouble*. London: Routledge.

Canguilhem G (1989) *The Normal and the Pathological*. New York: Zone Books.

Carter, S. (1995) 'Boundaries of danger and uncertainty: an analysis of the technological culture of risk assessment' in J. Gabe (ed.), *Medicine, Risk and Health*. Oxford: Blackwell.

Cixous, H. (1990) 'The laugh of the medusa' in R. Walder (ed.), *Literature in the Modern World*. Oxford: Oxford University Press.

Deleuze, G. and Guattari, F. (1984) *Anti-Oedipus: Capitalism and Schizophrenia*. London: Athlone.

Deleuze, G. and Guattari, F. (1988) *A Thousand Plateaus*. London: Athlone.

Department of the Environment (1995) *A Guide to Risk Assessment and Risk Management for Environmental Protection*. London: HMSO.

Derrida, J. (1976) *Of Grammatology*. Baltimore: Johns Hopkins.

De Swaan, A. (1990) *The Management of Normality*. London: Routledge.

Douglas, M. (1966) *Purity and Danger*. London: Routledge.

Douglas, M. (1973) *Natural Symbols*. Harmondsworth: Penguin.

Douglas, M. (1992) *Risk and Blame. Essays in Cultural Theory*. London: Routledge.

Foucault, M. (1970) *The Order of Things*. London: Tavistock.

Foucault, M. (1980) 'Truth and power' in C. Gordon (ed.), *Power/knowledge*. Brighton: Harvester Press.

Foucault, M. (1981) *The History of Sexuality*. Vol 1: *An Introduction*. Harmondsworth: Penguin.

Fox, N.J. (1991) 'Postmodernism, rationality and the evaluation of health care'. *Sociological Review*. **39**(4) 709–44.

Fox, N.J. (1992) *The Social Meaning of Surgery.* Buckingham: Open University Press.

Fox, N.J. (1993) *Postmodernism, Sociology and Health.* Buckingham: Open University Press.

Fox, N.J. (1995) 'Postmodern perspectives on care: the vigil and the gift', *Critical Social Policy*, **15**: 107–25.

Fox, N.J. (1997a) 'The promise of postmodernism for the sociology of health and medicine' in G. Scambler and P. Higgs (eds), *Modernity, Medicine and Health.* London: Routledge.

Fox, N.J. (1997b) 'Is there life after Foucault? Texts, frames and differends' in A. Petersen and R. Bunton (eds), *Foucault, Health and Medicine.* London: Routledge.

Gabe, J. (ed.) (1995) *Medicine, Risk and Health.* Oxford: Blackwell.

Glassner, B. (1989) 'Fitness and the postmodern self', *Journal of Health and Social Behaviour*, **30**(2): 180–91.

Grinyer, A. (1995) 'Risk, the real world and naive sociology' in J. Gabe (ed.), *Medicine, Risk and Health.* Oxford: Blackwell.

Johnstone-Bryden, I.M. (1995) *Managing Risk.* Aldershot: Avebury.

Kelly, M. and Charlton, B. (1995) 'The modern and the postmodern in health promotion' in R. Bunton, S. Nettleton and R. Burrows (eds), *The Sociology of Health Promotion.* London: Routledge.

Lash, S. (1991) 'Genealogy and the body: Foucault/Deleuze/Nietzsche' in M. Featherstone, M. Hepworth and B.S. Turner (eds), *The Body.* London: Sage.

Lash, S. (1994) 'Reflexivity and its doubles: structures, aesthetics, community' in U. Beck, A. Giddens and S. Lash (eds), *Reflexive Modernization.* Cambridge: Polity.

London Hazards Centre (1993) *VDU Work and the Hazards to Health.* London: London Hazards Centre.

Ogden, J. (1995) 'Psychosocial theory and the creation of the risky self', *Social Science & Medicine*, **40**(3): 409–15.

Petersen, A.R. (1994) 'Governing images: media constructions of the "normal", "healthy" subject', *Media Information Australia*, **72** (May): 32–40.

Prior, L. (1995) 'Chance and modernity: accidents as a public health problem' in R. Bunton, S. Nettleton and R. Burrows (eds), *The Sociology of Health Promotion.* London: Routledge

Rayner, S. (1992) 'Cultural theory and risk analysis' in S. Krimsky and D. Golding (eds), *Social Theories of Risk.* Westport, CO: Praeger.

Rogers, R. and Salvage, J. (1988) *Nurses at Risk. A Guide to Health and Safety at Work.* London: Heinemann.

Sacks, O. (1985) *The Man who Mistook his Wife for a Hat.* London: Picador.

Sacks, O. (1991) *Awakenings.* London: Picador.

Sacks, O. (1995) *An Anthropologist on Mars: Seven Paradoxical Tales.* London: Picador.

Scott, S. and Freeman, R. (1995) 'Prevention as a problem of modernity: the example of HIV and AIDS' in J. Gabe (ed.), *Medicine, Risk and Health.* Oxford: Blackwell.

Sedgewick, P. (1982) *Psychopolitics.* London: Pluto.

Thorogood, N. (1995) '"London dentist in HIV scare": HIV and dentistry in popular discourse' in R. Bunton, S. Nettleton and R. Burrows (eds), *The Sociology of Health Promotion*. London: Routledge.

White, S. (1991) *Political Theory and Postmodernism*. Cambridge: Cambridge University Press.

WHO (1985) *Targets for Health for All*. Geneva: World Health Organisation.

Wright, W. (1982) *The Social Logic of Health*. New Brunswick: Rutgers University Press.

Wynne, B. (1992) 'Risk and social learning: reification to engagement' in S. Krimsky and D. Golding (eds), *Social Theories of Risk*. Westport, CO: Praeger.

12 Occupational Health Issues and Strategies: A View from Primary Health Care

Simon Pickvance

Continuing with the theme of political strategies to improve working conditions and health, the following chapter explores a number of policy areas from the vantage point of primary health care. It highlights the need for both local and global responses to problems of work-related ill health. At local level, primary health care offers a relatively underused source of support that could potentially enhance workers' knowledge and control. It could also offer a much needed independent source of information and advice on occupational health issues, outside of the employer dominated services that currently exist. While local responses are important, the global nature of occupational health problems is increasingly apparent and this necessitates international collaboration between all those involved in promoting health at work.

Introduction

In this chapter I shall look at five areas of occupational health and safety provision, arguing that major changes must occur in each if there is to be significant reduction in the burden of work-related ill health. My perspective is derived from 18 years' experience of working with the Sheffield Occupational Health Project (OHP). This is an occupational health service in primary health care which employs non-medical staff from a range of backgrounds including research, health promotion and trade union activity. The Sheffield project has been funded partly by the health authority and partly from GP contributions to provide an advice service to patients in 25 practices (a quarter of all GP practices in Sheffield). Patients are referred to the OHP by primary health care staff. Project workers also undertake opportunistic screening in waiting rooms in order to profile problems of work-related ill health.

Primary health care offers an exceptional vantage point for seeing the patterns and extent of occupational morbidity in a population. Ninety-five per cent of the UK population is registered with a general practitioner and most patients visit their doctor at least once within a three-year period. The primary health care setting also provides special opportunities for intervening to help patients to improve their working conditions, and to obtain compensation to which they may be entitled. Advising on job adaptation and the employment rights of patients with disabilities also fits comfortably within the advocacy role of primary health care workers.

Reports from the few practitioners currently advising patients in primary health care provide evidence of enormous unmet need for advice in the community. This is growing as the contemporary working environment poses threats to health that differ greatly from the perceived risks of 25 years ago. Problems have been compounded during the same period by economic and labour market policies which have encouraged insecurity at work at the same time as reducing employment protection and lowering levels of social security and compensation for industrial disease and injury. Hence, workers are often inhibited from complaining about conditions and employers face diminished incentives to invest in newer and potentially safer technologies or to provide rehabilitation for sick or injured workers. The experience of those involved in occupational health projects suggests that we need to find new ways of addressing the problems of these workers, particularly those in small firms, the self-employed, the unemployed and those in the informal sector; as well as the needs of minority ethnic workers, homeworkers and shift workers. The common element in the experience of these groups is that they have access to minimal occupational health services or none at all and that those provided place a low priority on prevention.

Preventing occupational illness

Work is a major cause of ill health. A recent study attributed 5 per cent of disability in industrialised countries to employment (Murray and Lopez, 1997). Yet most studies underestimate the impact of work on health, failing to elicit its contribution to some of the most common causes of illness, such as heart disease, and understating the prevalence of recognised occupational diseases (Association of British Insurers, 1996; European Foundation for the Improvement of Living and Working Conditions, 1996; Jones et al., 1998). Other problems such as stress-related illness are rarely recognised in occupational health statistics. Yet work-related stress is a growing problem and may well be one of the ways in which inequalities in society affect the health of whole populations (Wilkinson, 1996).

Occupational ill health is costly both in human and financial terms. In the UK the costs of work-related ill health have been estimated at roughly £11–16 billion per annum (Davies and Teasdale, 1993). Yet few workers have access to adequate prevention services. Economic developments and labour market policies have further undermined the development of occupational health services. In Sheffield, the local economy is increasingly dominated by small firms, employers with multiple premises, subcontracting and self-employment, and many workers and employers have no access to specialised prevention knowledge and skills inside the workplace. A Health and Safety Executive (HSE) report noted that only half the UK workforce has access to any occupational health professional via the workplace for any purpose whatsoever (Bunt, 1993).

Occupational health provision which does exist is often employer led. Hence services provided within the workplace are often more concerned with pre-employment screening and fitness for work than with a programme of planned prevention (Ballard, 1996). Alternative modes of provision, such as those being developed within primary health care offer advantages to both workers and employers that are yet to be widely appreciated (Pickvance, 1992; Rasanen et al., 1993). The expansion of independent multidisciplinary occupational health services, some in primary health care, others contracting directly to employers, would allow many more workers to gain access to knowledge and skills including advocacy, rehabilitation and welfare rights, as well as occupational psychology and ergonomics. These are particularly important given the growth of the insecure workforce (Brewster et al., 1997) and changing patterns of occupational risk (see Daykin, this volume).

Prevention of occupational disease is one of the aims of health and safety legislation and enforcement activity in industrial societies. Falls in the incidence of compensatable diseases in these societies are often taken as evidence of the effectiveness of such activities in preventing work-related ill health. Yet the impact of legislation may be complex, and the relative effectiveness of different ways of improving conditions at work has rarely been studied. Protective measures can in fact be introduced without any change in legislation and many agencies and organisations can contribute to prevention work.

The potential contribution of primary care-based occupational health projects to the prevention of work-related disease can be illustrated by means of the following example. In the mid-1980s Dave Gee, then Safety Officer for the General Municipal and Boilermakers Trade Union, contacted Sheffield's Trade Union Safety Committee (TUSC), to ask whether there was any evidence that hard metal disease, due to exposure to cobalt dust in the engineering and tool making industries, occurred in Sheffield. TUSC contacted Sheffield Occupational Health Project, whose advisers were able to examine routine data in order to identify patients whose exposure to cobalt dust had been recorded and check this information against their medical notes. This showed that there were indeed cases of hard metal disease in these general practice populations.

This exercise was followed by a media campaign at local and national levels. This in turn led to activity on the part of trade unions, trade associations, the Health and Safety Executive and solicitors. Although general legislation on the protection of workers from exposure to harmful substances existed prior to this in the form of the 1974 Health and Safety at Work etc. Act, little action had been taken. According to the manager of a Sheffield engineering firm, attitudes to use of hard metal (in tool tips) in local firms changed within a few months as a result of the publicity (personal communication).

Hence, even where legislation does exist, there is no guarantee that this will lead to effective prevention. Employers can evade implementation and, in the case of EU Directives, member states themselves can interpret directives in different ways. The 1992 EU Framework Directive on Management of Health and Safety at Work for example required employers to introduce comprehensive services. In some member states, this was interpreted in relation to the demands of the International Labour Organisation Convention and Recommendation 161 and 171 (ILO, 1985; Vogel, 1993). This called for the development of multidisciplinary occupational health services and emphasised the social and not just the physical aspects of workplace health. It prioritised prevention over other functions of workplace health provision and, importantly, called for the independence of occupational health services from employers.

By contrast, the UK government has adopted a more limited approach, concentrating on risk assessment and turning it into a management function. Assessment of the need for specialist prevention services is left to 'competent persons' in the management structure. Yet this form of risk assessment can often amount to little more than a bureaucratic procedure.

Legislation for the control of work hazards is only useful if it can be translated into action by managers and workers. Research into effective safety management has shown that the involvement of the whole workforce through safety representatives and joint safety committees produces the greatest reductions in accidents (Reilly et al., 1995). Innovation in prevention methods is best carried out as a participatory process involving everyone in the workplace (Gustavsen et al., 1996).

Research shows that workers' control over certain aspects of their work is a key influence on many common work-related health problems, including sick building syndrome, heart disease and musculoskeletal disorders (Karasek and Theorell, 1990). Further, increasing the control workers have in the workplace can in itself reduce occupational morbidity, as evidenced by physiological markers, sickness absence records and subjective reports (Karasek and Theorell, 1990). While the need for workers' participation is acknowledged in some areas, such as ergonomics, the need for workers to participate in risk assessment and safety management is only beginning to be more widely accepted (Trade Union Technical Bureau, 1995).

Research has also demonstrated the benefits of workers' participation in other areas of prevention work including the management of health and safety and occupational health services within an enterprise (Aldrich, 1993), and the devising of new working practices (Gustavsen et al., 1996; Moir and Buchholz, 1996).

Regulation and enforcement

While occupational health regulation is, at least in Europe, increasingly international, local variations in policy and ideology can have a significant impact. Under the Conservative administrations of the 1980s and 1990s Britain developed its own particular response to European legislation, characterised by government reluctance to transpose EU directives into local regulations. This lent credibility to employers' strategy of delaying compliance by asking for further clarification of what was required of them. These responses were underlined by a philosophy of deregulation, vigorously promoted by government, although never openly supported by more than a few employers (Department of Trade and Industry, 1994; Health and Safety Commission, 1994). These trends have had a lasting impact on regulation and enforcement activity. For example, the funding and effectiveness of enforcement agencies has been systematically reduced, further undermining the effectiveness of EU-inspired law (Institute of Professionals, Managers and Specialists, 1992). The role of the HSE has shifted from one of enforcement towards that of advice giving. At the same time, the shift in the economy towards smaller employment units has made even an advisory role increasingly difficult.

The processes of regulation, enforcement and compliance are complex and a number of agencies, including manufacturers, insurers and the media, may be involved as well as official enforcement agencies and employers. In the case of the EU 1992 Display Screen Equipment Directive, for instance, the UK the Health and Safety Executive let it be known that enforcement of the Display Screen Regulations would be a very low priority in its work. Yet there has been a dramatic change in the design of VDU workstations since the regulations appeared because computer manufacturers rather than employers responded to the requirements. The rapid turnover of office equipment meant that within a few years the design of VDU workstations (and to a lesser extent VDU tasks) was significantly altered (Breidensjo *et al.*, 1996).

While the influence of traditional enforcement agencies has diminished, other agencies have, sometimes unexpectedly, begun to assume an enforcement role. The fear generated by highly publicised cases of litigation over repetitive strain injuries among VDU workers appears to have influenced some employers even though much of this litigation is in fact unsuccessful. Indeed, increases in claims for civil damages have encouraged some insurance companies to act as enforcers, guiding their clients on what is likely to be considered negligent should they be sued.

The role of insurance companies in regulation and enforcement is, however, extremely problematic. They could certainly provide financial incentives to employers for effective health and safety management, offering what is potentially a more sensitive system for achieving compliance with standards. However, any such effects are likely to be short lived, since their efforts would probably be undermined by competitors offering insurance at lower prices (Boleat, 1996).

The media can also exert a powerful influence on attitudes to regulation and compliance. In 1977 a film called *Alice, the Fight for Life* was shown on television. Alice was a victim of asbestos-related disease. The programme changed the way in which asbestos was seen by hundreds of thousands of workers, with attitudes in the building trade in Sheffield changing overnight. It is at the time of writing still possible to buy asbestos in Sheffield for use, but that media event twenty years ago made more of a difference to the risks faced by workers than the Asbestos Regulations and the publication of guidance materials since 1969.

In summary, enforcement agencies alone cannot ensure compliance with every requirement of the law everywhere. Change does not occur as soon as law is passed; indeed it often precedes the law. When change does occur it may be the media, or trade unions, or trade associations, or manufacturers or enforcement agencies or several of these acting in concert which play the leading role. Like prevention, the effectiveness of regulation is influenced by the core values of society which give each institution its mandate to act. It is not, after all, the Scandinavian Labour Inspectorates which have been particularly esteemed by occupational health specialists throughout the world, but the Scandinavian social compact, which has been reflected in activities in the workplace and in the value society has attached to each of its health and safety institutions.

Workers' views on the future role of enforcement have varied during the 1990s. Some voices from the British labour movement have called for restoration and strengthening of enforcement agencies (Institute of Professionals, Managers and Specialists, 1992). Others have called for stronger disincentives to be applied (Hazards Campaign, 1996). Hence, there has been pressure to increase penalties on employers who are caught in breach of the law and to introduce new offences where employers' actions lead to the death of an employee. These arguments are strengthened by the fact that an increase in state regulation seems unlikely at the present time. Further, the proliferation of small firms is likely to defeat even a much enlarged enforcement agency's attempts to inspect every workplace regularly. The fear of severe penalties might, however, make employers police themselves and there is evidence that increasing the penalties for infringements of the law are at least as effective as increasing the frequency of inspectors' visits in raising standards (Hunt, 1995).

Most policy discussions on how to achieve compliance emphasise the importance of governmental agencies and the sanctions at their disposal. Few consider the system of negotiations and the sanctions available within every workplace: the role of active worker participation in health and safety management. In the UK, the 1978 Safety Representative Regulations gave trade union representatives a legally defined role in the management of health and safety. In Sheffield, trade union safety representatives are frequent users of the Occupational Health Project, requesting information and sometimes bringing groups of workers along for hearing or lung function tests where occupational damage is suspected. All reports on the activities of safety representatives have shown their effectiveness in lowering accident rates, in exposing the weaknesses of employers' safety management systems, and uncovering health problems (Dawson et al., 1988).

The EU Framework Directive and the UK Health and Safety (Consultation with Employees) Regulations 1996 have extended some of these representation rights to unorganised workplaces. However, this is only a small step in the development of participatory structures. The new health hazards of the 1980s and 1990s require a strengthening of the rights of health and safety representatives and an expansion of their role. They need to be able to influence all decisions affecting health and working conditions including those on management and investment.

Rehabilitation

Prior to the 1980s Sheffield steelworkers who had been injured at work or had breathing or heart problems might be kept on at work in lighter jobs until well into their sixties. However, the mass redundancies of the 1980s saw workers with activity-limiting health problems encouraged to take redundancy or offered early ill-health retirement. Apart from a small payment for their occupational deafness there has been no compensation for the long-term health problems they suffered – often chest disease caused by a mixture of steelworks dust, cigarette smoke and East End air. Instead of receiving programmes of retraining and job adaptation to mitigate these effects the long-term sick have been subjected to policies which imply that their situation is of their own, not society's, making. Hence claimants trying to obtain the long-term state ill-health benefit known as Incapacity Benefit will be denied support unless they pass a stringent test, even if there is no suitable work available locally.

Occupational health problems are societal problems although provision of employment for sufferers is usually left to individual employers. The failings of employers' occupational health services are perhaps most strongly apparent in relation to sick workers. The fitness of workers for the job they do is of paramount importance to employers in the lean economy of the 1990s. Hence occupational health services at work are closely concerned with pre-employment screening, with sickness absence monitoring, and with ill-health retirement and redundancy. The unforeseen impact of the repeated fitness screening of the labour force is that the workforce is fitter than its peers who are out of work. This places increased pressure on pension schemes and on social security spending on the long-term sick.

These trends have provided the context for the work of the occupational health projects (OHPs) in primary care. In addition to their traditional prevention role, project workers have increasingly become involved in rehabilitation issues, helping workers to find ways of making changes to their jobs or working environments so that they can carry on in employment. The alternative for these workers is often dismissal as their employment protection rights are severely limited. Hence the occupational health projects have also extended their activities to those out of work, advising on their entitlement to state benefits, compensation and pensions.

There are further collective consequences of increased health selection in the workplace. By studying the health of those who remain in employment, researchers have found that even in the most dangerous working environments, work appears to be health enhancing. The witnesses to the long-term effects of work on health are in reality to be encountered in the community and not in the workplace. This is why occupational health research in primary health care settings is important. Yet it remains sparse. In an attempt to fill the gap, Sheffield OHP has carried out a number of studies, including a follow-up of the long-term health problems of former steel workers which was carried out in collaboration with the Office of National Statistics (Sheffield Occupational Health Project, 1998).

While the picture appears bleak, there are trends which offer limited hope to workers. For example, sick workers are expensive to insurers as well as to governments. If an occupational accident or disease is the pretext for exclusion from the workforce the insurer, private or state will have to pick up the costs. In response to this, employers' liability insurers in many countries have attempted to force their clients to rehabilitate workers to reduce the compensation bill for lost wages (Pickvance, 1997).

Perhaps more hope can be drawn from increasing demands in the European Union and North America for an end to discrimination against disabled people. In the UK the introduction of the Disability Discrimination Act 1995 has encouraged employers to make reasonable adaptations to the workplace and to work requirements for employees with disabilities, and they must not discriminate against workers with disabilities at recruitment. However, the law, which carried forward European Union initiatives on disabilities, was out of kilter with the employment policies of Tory administrations. Like other recent EU-inspired advances in employment legislation in the UK it has been left as unenforceable as possible. There is at the time of writing no agency charged with enforcing the DDA and those who end up outside the workforce as a result of discrimination at work must go to a tribunal to prove their case.

Nevertheless the DDA does give a glimpse of what a humane policy towards people of working age with disabilities might be (see Pinder, this volume). It recognises that employers' interests can run counter to those of society as a whole. Employers shift the costs of making workers ill on to society when they exclude people of working age with work-related ill health from productive employment. This inevitably produces unfairness. Individual employers act in their own interest to make their own decisions about the level of fitness they require of their workforce. Governments, by the same token, must make consistent decisions about the criteria they adopt when paying out sickness-related benefits. Many people fall between these patterns of exclusion and inclusion, effectively excluded from available work in their area, and yet not included in the uniform requirements of illness-related social security.

Some societies place a high priority on the development of the working capacities of all those of working age, whether they have a health problem or not. However, no society has achieved a continuous process of adaptation of work to the worker and of workers of all ages to the new requirements of work (see however Finnish Institute of Occupational Health, 1996). In a review of occupational health in Sweden, the National Institute of Working Life found that employees with disabilities were concentrated in jobs where they had least control over their work, and where they were at greater risk to their health than workers without disabilities (Jarvholm, 1996).

In the context of global trade, cheap manual labour and data processing, the postindustrialised societies will depend more and more upon knowledge-based employment and work requiring specifically human creativity and sensitivity. The rehabilitation challenges of the future will focus, on the one hand, on the socially excluded sectors of the workforce experienced only in manual work and unable to do even that, and, on the other, on psychological casualties of work, damaged by psychological burnout and the physiological consequences of psychosocial stress.

Compensation

Compensation systems for industrial diseases and injuries are in crisis all over the world. The UK Labour Force Survey showed that workers perceived the extent of work-related ill health as many times (for some diseases hundreds of times) higher than the total number of cases compensated by the state and employers' liability insurers (Hodgson *et al.*, 1993; Jones *et al.*, 1998). Most compensation systems fail in some way to cope with the most common or newer occupational health problems, such as musculoskeletal disorders and stress. Some, for example the Dutch state system, do not distinguish between ill health caused by work and illness from other causes. Others are run almost completely by private insurers, albeit on terms dictated largely by state legislation.

The UK is unusual among the older industrialised countries in having two unsatisfactory systems rather than one. The state system compensates 2500 new cases of 67 different occupational diseases each year. The private system pays out roughly the same amount of money as the state system for a very much larger number of claims, and for a wider range of illnesses. Hence, while compensating far more victims, the private system makes on average, much smaller awards. In the UK, a recent HSE publication (Davies and Teasdale, 1993) showed another reason why the workers' dissatisfaction with these systems is so great: insurance only covers a relatively small part of the costs of occupational illness and injury. There are many hidden uninsured costs borne by the victim.

The two systems of compensation and the relationships between them are deeply flawed. The DSS system awards compensation for 67 'prescribed diseases', many of which no longer occur in the UK. Ten diseases account for 90 per cent of claims, and yet the commonest work-related conditions reported in the Labour Force Survey are not among them (Hodgson *et al.*, 1993). The process of adding to the list of diseases is ultimately constrained by cash limits. Most occupational diseases on the EU's list are absent or not fully included in the DSS list, despite the authoritative status of the EU list which was drawn up by a group of leading specialists (European Commission, 1994). By way of response to the increased demands on the DSS Industrial Injuries Scheme, Tory administrations successively cut entitlement to benefits while also reducing levels of payment to those (few) entitled to compensation. Latterly there were even threats to the continued existence of the state system of industrial injuries compensation as a whole.

The common law/damages system depends for its efficacy upon the access plaintiffs have to civil justice, and upon the even-handedness of the legal process. But most workers and ex-workers are excluded because they cannot afford the risk of paying legal costs if they lose their case. Workers are all too often represented by relatively inexperienced solicitors and witnesses. Faced with a comparatively coherent defence on the part of insurers, they are reluctant to risk their savings in a David and Goliath contest. No-fault compensation systems, where they exist, offer a less strenuous route to compensation. However, payments under such schemes are often very low.

Sick and injured workers face the additional strain of negotiating their way through these complex compensation systems. This might be acceptable if between them the systems compensated for income losses and for pain and suffering in full. But when they do not, claimants' sense of injustice is redoubled.

All national systems of compensation face similar problems, but systems in some countries have gone much further to address the shortcomings experienced by claimants. For example, improving the rehabilitation services offered to victims both protects their future employment and reduces the need for compensation for lost income. In some countries insurance systems have linked compensation closely to prevention by relating premiums paid to claims made in an employment sector or by a given employer and by linking priority setting for prevention agencies to trends in claims. These strategies have yet to be developed in the UK.

Compensation systems can be made more equitable, but the scale of the mismatch between expectation and reality in most countries is such that reforms in other areas of occupational health policy are essential too. The lists of diseases compensated under no-fault schemes (whether run by the state or agreed between protagonists in civil disputes) need more accurately to reflect what workers see as the deleterious effects of work, and premiums should be raised to increase compensation awards. Ultimately, however, the only method of meeting needs more effectively lies outside the compensation system itself, in areas of employment policy, in support for research and in measures to improve the management of health and safety at work.

Research

There are two broad approaches to occupational health research. The reactive view suggests that research need only be undertaken once an occupational hazard has been identified. In contrast, the pre-emptive perspective suggests that research should be a constitutive part of any planned change to work processes. Throughout the 1980s and 1990s the UK approach has been at the *laissez-faire* and hence largely reactive end of this spectrum (Bacon, 1995).

A patient who recently sought advice from the Sheffield Occupational Health Project had rinsed sheets of stainless steel with a chlorinated solvent for twenty years. By the time he was made redundant his children had started to tease him for 'gurgy-burgling' – slipping into nonsensical speech without noticing. This dysphasia is one of a group of symptoms he exhibits which are typical of organic solvent encephalopathy. In Scandinavia, research over the past twenty years has deepened knowledge of this syndrome and led to a programme of solvent substitution, and the compensation and rehabilitation of sufferers. In contrast, research in UK into the effects of organic solvents on the central nervous system has been limited, with few contributions to the world literature on the subject.

In the period following the Second World War, occupational health research in the UK was given a higher priority, reflecting the prevailing mood of social reconstruction. Long-term support was provided for research on a number of industrial diseases including coal mine pneumoconiosis, chronic obstructive airways disease, cardiovascular disease and its connection with sedentary work, and for a time byssinosis – the lung disease of cotton workers. These projects put UK scientists at the forefront of knowledge in their fields and were closely tied to measures to improve working conditions (Schilling, 1998).

However, by the end of the 1970s funding of research into occupational health and safety by the HSE was just a few million pounds a year. Much of this funding was short-term contract research or related to the long-term commitment to safety in coal mines. These were the dying embers in the fire of a long-established research system in which experts with state support responded to the needs they identified. By the early 1990s long-term commitment to major research initiatives in occupational health was almost entirely absent in the UK. This picture is not unique: in Australia even deeper cuts in occupational research funding are being implemented, effectively bringing federal research spending in occupational health to an end.

Workers' needs can be spelt out quite simply; they need research which is pre-emptive, or at least quickly responsive to their problems. It should be of high quality and it should spell out the practical consequences of its conclusions. There should be effective mechanisms for involving workers in research and in disseminating results as well as developing practical solutions based on them.

Some research programmes in Europe have developed along these lines. For example, the Work Environment Funds in Scandinavian countries in the 1980s, and the programmes of the Nordic institutes for occupational health research have provided institutional routes by which workers and employers can influence research programmes. The European Coal and Steel Community's medical research programme has, built into its committee structure, opportunities for workers' representatives to make their preferences clear. A great deal of thought has been given to how research results affect reality (Gustavsen *et al.*, 1996); conferences debate the issue, and the European Union's Community Ergonomics programme has produced practical summary sheets on completed projects.

In the absence of such initiatives in the UK, research into occupational health and safety does go on. Some of it is commissioned by solicitors for groups of litigants, or by television companies who achieve changes in government policy in a haphazard way. At the same time, in hundreds of workplaces throughout UK workers have carried out their own research, developing the tradition of lay or workers' epidemiology (Watterson, 1994; Anon, 1995). There has been a long tradition of astute workers, as well as concerned occupational health professionals, drawing attention to clusters of cases of hitherto unrecognised occupational morbidity (Wegman, 1995). Lay epidemiology goes further than this, strengthening workers' cases for action on the patterns of ill health at work they uncover.

Workers' epidemiology has grown internationally from a few pioneering studies in the mid-1970s to become the normal way by which workers draw attention to patterns of work-related ill health in their workplaces (Loewenson *et al.*, 1994, and this volume). It is, by definition, responsive to workers' needs. It provides a challenge to employer-led risk assessments such as those implemented in response to EU Directives. In addition, since the results are owned collectively by workers themselves, it has a good chance of bridging the gap between research and practical changes in work processes.

Workers' epidemiology does have its weaknesses however. For example, it tends to be specific to a particular workplace or process so that the benefits are not always easily generalised. In Sheffield the

Occupational Health Project plays a key role in supporting workers' epidemiology, providing independent advice, information, literature and support for the development of methods of data collection and analysis that are both sensitive and robust.

A gap exists between what the shrinking community of occupational health researchers and the growing band of worker epidemiologists can do and what is required. One response would be to admit defeat – to accept that some nations, including the UK, would in future be clients, translating the findings of the research establishments of other countries. This would not sit easily with the proven value of local participation in addressing research questions. While there is a need for more research to be organised on an international level in response to globalisation, local institutions are also needed. These should draw on the responsiveness of workers' epidemiology and investigate ways of increasing the applicability of its conclusions.

Conclusion

This chapter has examined five areas of occupational health policy from a vantage point within primary health care. Concerted action in all of these areas is needed to improve health and safety at work in the long term. This chapter has also explored the links between these policy areas. Insurers can act as enforcers and workers as researchers, while enforcers cannot achieve compliance without effective prevention services. Ideally these should help with rehabilitation of sick and injured workers into employment. Rehabilitation reduces the need for compensation, while compensation systems require sound research to predict future risks. A common feature of the changes which are needed in each area is the need for less hierarchical, more participatory structures, which involve workers as advisers, researchers and managers of workplace change.

However, given the deep changes to the structure of the economy which have occurred during the last twenty years, even these developments may be insufficient to protect the health of the workforce in the future. This period has seen the most dramatic changes in the nature of work since the rise of mass employment in manufacturing in the nineteenth century. The next twenty years may see even greater changes. Hundreds of thousands of jobs which are now done in workplaces could with existing technology be performed at home. Activities which were once mainly performed by unpaid carers in the household, such as looking after elderly people, have increasingly taken the form of paid employment. At the same time, the refusal of governments to countenance increased social provision is shifting some traditional caring back to the household as unpaid work.

Changes in the nature of work and the rapid pace of globalisation require rapidly responding structures in occupational health, but these must be structures that workers can influence. The need for a truly international labour movement networking to achieve common standards is being widely felt (*Workers' Health International Newsletter*, 1996). This movement needs to build alliances with the influential consumer movements which are starting to emerge in some countries. The alternative is a globalised economy which will sink towards the lowest standards of worker protection.

References

Anon (1995) 'Safety representatives survey', *Hazards Bulletin*, **52**: 8–9.
Aldrich, P. (1993) *Report on the Danish Occupational Health Services.* Brussels: Trade Union Technical Bureau.
Association of British Insurers (1996) *Statistics Bulletin 1995 Results.* London: ABI.
Bacon, J. (1995) 'Occupational health: the next 50 years.' *The 1995 Lane Lecture*, 15 November, Centre for Occupational Health, University of Manchester.
Ballard, J. (1996). 'Occupational health nurses: an OHR survey', *Occupational Health Review*, **59**: 1–8 and **60**: 21–17.
Boleat, M. (1996) Paper delivered at the TUC Conference on preventing injury and ill-health: the role of insurance, December 1996.
Breidensjo, M., Bolvie, P.-E. and Gustafsson, S. (1996) *Evaluation of the Introduction of the EEC Display Screen Equipment Directive in Sweden.* Sweden: TCO.
Brewster, C., Mayne, L. and Tregarskis, O. (1997) 'Flexible working in Europe: a review of the evidence', *Management International Review*, Special Issue 1997/1: 85–103.
Bunt, K. (1993) *Occupational Health Provision at Work, Contract Research Report 57*, Health and Safety Executive. London: HMSO.
Davies, N.V. and Teasdale, P. (1993) *The Costs to the British Economy of Work Accidents and Work-related Ill Health.* London: HSE Books.
Dawson, W., Willman, P., Bamford, M. and Clinton, A. (1988) *Safety at Work: The Limits of Self-regulation.* Cambridge: Cambridge University Press.
Department of Trade and Industry (1994) *Deregulation – Cutting Red Tape.* London: DTI.
European Commission Directorate for General Employment, Industrial Relations and Social Affairs (1994) *Information Notices on Diagnosis of Occupational Diseases.* (EUR 14768 EN). Luxembourg: European Commission.

European Foundation for the Improvement of Living and Working Conditions (1996) *Second European Survey on Working Conditions*. Dublin: European Foundation for the Improvement of Living and Working Conditions.

Finnish Institute of Occupational Health (1997) *Work Health and Safety*. Helsinki: FIOH.

Gustavsen, B., Hofmaier, B., Ekman, Philips, M. and Wikman, A. (1996) *Concept-driven Development and the Organisation of the Process of Change*. Amsterdam: J. Benjamin.

Hazards Campaign (1996) *Health and Safety Charter*. Bradford: Hazards Campaign.

Health and Safety Commission (1994) *Review of Regulation: Main Report*. London: HMSO.

Hodgson, J.T., Jones, J.R., Elliott, R.C. and Osman, J. (1993) *Self-reported Work-related Illness*, Research Paper 33. London: HMSO.

Hunt, G. (1995) *Michigan Disability Prevention Study – Research Highlights*. Kalamazoo, Michigan: WE Upjohn Institute of Employment Research.

Institute of Professionals Managers and Specialists (1992) *Health and Safety: An Alternative Report*. London: IPMS.

International Labour Organisation (1985) *Convention and Recommendation concerning Occupational Health Services. Convention 161 and Recommendation 171*. Geneva: ILO.

Jarvholm, B. (ed.) (1996) *Working Life and Health: A Swedish Survey*. Sweden: National Institute for Working Life.

Jones, J.R., Hodgson, J.T., Clegg, T.A. and Elliott, R.C. (1998) *Self-reported Work-related Illness in 1995*. London: Government Statistical Service.

Karasek, R. and Theorell, T. (1990) *Healthy Work; Stress, Productivity and the Transformation of Working Life*. New York: Basic Books.

Loewenson, R., Laurell, A.C. and Hogstedt, C. (1994) *Participatory Approaches in Occupational Health Research, Arbete och Halsa*, **38**: 1–60.

Moir, S. and Buchholz, B. (1996) 'Emerging participatory approaches to ergonomic interventions in the construction industry,' *Amer. J. Ind. Med.* **29**: 425–30.

Murray, C.J.L. and Lopez, A.D. (1997) 'Global mortality, disability and the contribution of risk factors: Global Burden of Disease Study', *The Lancet*, **349**: 1436–42.

National Occupational Health Forum (1997) *Consensus Statement*. London: NOHF.

Pickvance, S. (1992) 'An occupational health service in primary care', *Occup. Med.*, **42**: 61–3

Pickvance, S. (1997) 'Employers' liability: a system out of balance', *Occupational Health Review*, November/December 1997: 10–13.

Rasanen, K., Notkola, V., Kankaanpaa, H., Peurala, M. and Husman, K. (1993) 'Role of occupational health services as a part of illness-related primary care in Finland', *Occup. Med.* **43**(1) Suppl. 1: S23–S27.

Reilly, B., Paci, P. and Holl, P. (1995) 'Unions, safety committees and workplace injuries', *Brit. J Ind. Rel.*, **33**(2): 275–88.

Schilling, R.S.F. (1998) *A Challenging Life*. London: Canning Press.

Sheffield Occupational Health Project (1998) *Report 1996–8*. Sheffield: SOHP.

Trade Union Technical Bureau (1995) *Risk Assessment*. Brussels: TUTB.

Vogel, L. (1993) Prevention at the workplace: an initial review of how the 1989 Community framework Directive is being implemented. Brussels: European Trade Union Technical Bureau.

Watterson, A. (1994) 'Whither lay epidemiology in UK? Public health in policy and practice', *J. Public Health Medicine*, **16**(3).

Wegman, D.H. (1995) 'Investigations into the use of symptom reports for studying toxic epidemics', *New Epidemics in Occupational Health*, Helsinki: Finnish Institute of Occupational Health.

Wilkinson, R.G. (1996) *Unhealthy Societies*. London: Routledge.

Workers Health International Newsletter (1996) *International Directory of Worker Health and Safety Contacts*. Sheffield: Hazards Publications.

13 PARTICIPATORY APPROACHES IN OCCUPATIONAL HEALTH RESEARCH

Rene Loewenson, Asa C. Laurell and
Christer Hogstedt

Several of the contributors to this volume have noted the growing interest in more participatory methods of health and social research. This chapter explores these methods in more depth, highlighting ways in which in the workplace in particular the traditional divide between the 'experts' and the subjects of research is beginning to be challenged. The implications of these new approaches are explored through an examination of studies undertaken in Europe, Africa and Latin America. The authors identify settings where health and safety professionals collaborate with workers' representatives to ensure that the research being undertaken is relevant to their needs and interests. They also outline a more radical approach where traditional modes of scientific endeavour are challenged and workers themselves are given a more active role in occupational health research and in the development of policies to promote healthier workplaces.

Introduction

Research is a process through which new knowledge and understanding is generated with the aim of achieving change. Why should participation be an issue in this process, and what impact does it have on the nature of the knowledge and its usefulness for change? This chapter explores the general concept of participation in occupational health, and then the issues in and forms of participatory research (PR) approaches in occupational health. Finally, it examines whether participatory research in occupational health produces new knowledge that is scientific and leads to change. It is not the aim of this chapter to argue that participatory approaches have an exclusive or superior role in generating new occupational health knowledge and practice, but that they may be more appropriate and effective than non participatory approaches in certain circumstances.

Participatory approaches in occupational health

Work is a product of the form and level of development of the labour process and of the social relations of production. It is the interaction between the two which determines the health profile of workers (and their community) (Wintersberger, 1985), and even further, the extent to which work-related ill health is recognised (Ramirez et al., 1985). In the twentieth century work processes have changed at a rapid pace leading to new forms of production, of work and of work organisation, with complex systems involving highly specialised inputs. In the early twentieth century advances in technology were generally made within regimented production systems involving centralised decision making over the work process. While tripartite structures existed to manage the potentially conflictual interests in production, these did not necessarily challenge management control of the technical process of production. In more recent decades there has been a shift in both the expectations of workers and in the organisation of work towards creating greater levels of worker participation in solving problems and making decisions in the work process (Noro et al., 1991).

Struggles for democratisation of working life in many parts of the world, north and south, have challenged the assumption that change should be a product of technical proficiency and knowledge implemented through decisions by high level policy makers and the technocrats that guide them. Swedish working life research in the 1970s was informed by the view that production systems should reflect social goals of democratic working life, including workers' control of the pace and working methods (Gardell, 1982; Johnson and Johansson, 1991). The research demonstrated that machine pacing, isolation, piece rate pay, and authoritarian management systems had negative social and psychological consequences for working people (Johnson and Johansson, 1991). To add economic impetus, the impact of quality control circles on the productivity and competitive advantage of Japanese companies led to a closer examination in many countries of the role and impact of worker participation in the organisation of work as a critical factor in determining productivity, work satisfaction and competitiveness (Noro *et al.*, 1991).

Such trends towards increased participation confront equally powerful trends that can and often do undermine participation, such as in the separation of the component parts of production across different continents and the hierarchies of decision making in transnational production or in the economic conditions that create conflict over production.

In occupational health (OH) in the past few decades there has also been a progressive shift in approach, in law and in practice that reflects a more central role for those who experience the hazards in knowing about, acting on, regulating and making decisions about the production processes that affect them (Ramirez *et al.*, 1985). This partly draws from the recognition that workers are closest to and thus most familiar with the work process and hence the desire to locate preventive action as close to the shop floor as possible (Wintersberger, 1985). It recognises the important role for the experience and perceptions of those at the shop floor as an input to understanding workplace hazards and work-related health, in reflecting the ecological interaction of workplace hazards and in enabling realistic occupational health interventions in small and medium enterprises (Gustavsen, 1985; Kogi, 1991; Noro *et al.*, 1991). It also draws to varying degrees from recognition of the potential conflict of interests at the workplace, and thus the need for workers to protect their interests. Such participation has taken various forms: from consultation to co-determination, from indirect delegated formal 'representative' tripartite structures to direct involvement of shop floor workers, individually or collectively. Such participatory occupational health approaches may also confront or transform management norms in production.

Participatory research in occupational health

While the understanding of how work affects health has grown rapidly in this century, it has still been outstripped by the pace of change in industrial processes. Knowledge on occupational health has also not been matched by health interventions in either rich and poor countries (Noweir, 1986; Oleru *et al.*, 1990; Wegman and Fine, 1990). Hence there continues to be a need to develop work on the relationships

between exposures and health effects, on occupational health interventions and on the factors that affect the application of occupational
health knowledge (Wegman and Fine, 1990). In underdeveloped countries, there is an additional pressure for research to expose the patterns
of occupational injury and illness not identified by inadequate route-
reporting systems and not socially recognised.

There are debates about *how* this new knowledge in occupational
health is generated. Democratisation within society has brought scientific knowledge increasingly within the public and popular domain, at
a time when the complexity of many scientific disciplines has, in fact,
alienated the potential beneficiaries. In the often conflictual conditions
of the workplace, access to knowledge and information has been recognised as a critical basis for effective participation. Hence, in 1981, a
Swedish Trade Union report on research policy noted that the ability of
trade unions to influence occupational health depended on the degree
to which they were able to determine the questions or problems that
were the object of occupational health research and to bring scientific
resources to bear on these questions (Ostberg *et al.*, 1991).

Involvement in and control of the research process

The demand by workers or their representative organisations for
greater control of the research agenda and process has led to participatory processes that have involved the affected community (generally
the workers) in the design, implementation, analysis and interpretation of the data and/or use of the results for action. The increased
complexity of working life, the need to access shop floor knowledge of
work and organisational processes, increased emphasis on stress and
other subjectively experienced conditions, the increasing recognition of
multifactorial illness and the need to determine illness in early stages
has motivated a greater recognition of the subjective experience and
the involvement of workers as central to inquiry and intervention
(Foot-Whyte, 1983; Gustavsen, 1985; Raimondi, 1985). Such participatory research approaches have been used:

- to expose unrecognised levels of work-related illness
- to study subjective symptoms in an effective way
- to measure exposure and outcomes without high cost
  technology/skills
- to increase worker capacity and involvement

- to give greater attention to cognitive, knowledge and experience of workers in identifying analysing and solving ergonomic problems (Garrigou *et al.*, 1995)
- to enhance the potential for action outcomes from the research findings.

One example of such a shift in control of both the research agenda and process occurred in Sweden, where there has been a highly unionized working class with substantial political power and well established mechanisms for institutional collective bargaining (Martin, 1992). Structural change in the economy in the late 1960s imposed costs on workers of labour displacement, intensified work and reduced quality of the work environment. Between 1968 and 1980, the Swedish Trade Union Congress (LO) carried out three surveys of its members to obtain a comprehensive picture of the reported physical hazards in the work environment and the health impact on workers; to examine psychosocial hazards and their impact on work-related stress and, in 1980, to explore changes in work environments and workers' health over the decade. LO employed professionals to construct and analyse the questionnaires in these surveys but kept control of the research process. Participation in this research thus remained at the level of the union, reflecting partly the system of consensus and centralised collective bargaining in Sweden. The use of members' reported assessments introduced potential bias but also provided a strong mandate for union negotiations using the data. The first surveys contributed to greater attention, programmes and resources being directed towards the working environment, backed by new laws and resources for work environment research through the Work Environment Fund (Loewenson *et al.*, 1994).

In Zimbabwe, a similar union-controlled research project was carried out under the more conflictual environment of economic underdevelopment. In such conditions, low profitability and low value-added production yields a level of employer resistance to occupational health liabilities and official assessments underreport occupational injury and illness (Zwi *et al.*, 1988; Kouabenan, 1990). Combined with the scarcity of professionals, this situation has led to pragmatic initiatives to simplify research techniques and measurement tools to allow for greater worker participation (Alakija, 1981; Hessel and Sluis-Cremer, 1985; Fonn *et al.*, 1988).

In 1989 when the Zimbabwe Congress of Trade Unions established a health department, one of the authors, worker researchers and medical students prepared an assessment of the current occupational health situation from reported data. When this was discussed by union leadership it exposed a gap between workers' experiences in the workplace and the reported patterns of injury and illness, and between workers' health needs and union collective bargaining agreements. This motivated a second union-based research activity, which, in a series of surveys over a two-year period, described the profile of work environments and occupational health practices. Unionists responsible for health and safety and later shop floor worker representatives collected the reported information from management, workers' representatives and workers. The profile of hazards was compiled from workers' subjective perceptions, from checklists completed by unions and from occupational hygiene measurements. The results of these surveys were used by unions at workplace, industry and national level to negotiate changes in workplace organisation on health and safety and recognition of worker health and safety representatives, to identify and discuss key problems to be addressed at workplace level and to raise the profile of occupational health problems experienced by workers. The research increased capacity in the unions to intervene in occupational health policy and programmes and made workers more confident to raise and debate technical issues in occupational health (Zimbabwe Congress of Trade Unions, 1992, 1994).

In these forms of participatory research the traditional scientific method is shared with worker participants, the researcher retains the role of expert, but facilitates the use and understanding of this expertise towards questions defined by the subjects. This enables more direct and informed action and exposes new occupational health problems for further scientific study. In the Zimbabwean and Swedish studies, as in many examples of PR work, the 'participation' and control by shop floor workers is indirect, being delegated to representative structures such as unions.

New approaches to the conceptualisation of knowledge

There is however a second and deeper basis to some participatory research approaches that conceptualises the production of knowledge as itself an outcome of social relations. Hence, it is asserted that popular systems of knowledge have existed in parallel with the dominant system throughout history, such as in traditional health systems, in the knowledge aimed at basic survival and in the collective social perceptions of reality of the poor. However, these systems have been largely unrecognised and neglected unless asserted by the pressure of social organisation (Fals-Borda, 1987; Tandon, 1988). This has generated a demand for a process of inquiry that recognises and organises the knowledge of ordinary people and that challenges the kind of 'expert knowledge' that suppresses or marginalises as unimportant the experience of the majority (Tandon, 1988). Implicitly, the generation of such knowledge cannot be delegated. Subjective experience is not interpreted as bias and controlled, for is primary and is validated through collective consensus (Misti *et al.*, 1983). With the increasing awareness of complex multifactorial causal models, 'subjectivity' and collective experience are proposed as one means towards a holistic model of reality that inherently involve multiple factors and outcomes (Misti *et al.*, 1983; Fals-Borda and Rahman, 1991; Frideres, 1992).

One of the most significant experiences of this form of participatory research on work-related health is that which developed in Italy in the mid-1960s. The Italian Workers' Model (WM) was originally developed by workers and union activists at a Fiat factory, supported by professionals and students (Berlinguer, 1977). The upsurge in labour movement activity in 1969, involving millions of workers, led to the application of the Workers' Model (WM) in workplaces across the country (Grisoni and Portelli, 1972; Laurell, 1984).

The Workers' Model (WM) organised the hazards/loads of the work environment into four 'risk groups':

1. those present inside and outside the workplace, for example noise, temperature
2. those typical of the workplace, for example dust, gases, vapours, radiations
3. those that produce physical fatigue
4. those that provoke mental fatigue.

These risk groups corresponded to workers' experience and perception of the work environment and enabled a 'common language' between workers and professionals. The principle of no-delegation made the main subjects of the studies rank and file workers and not their representatives or the professionals. The research was based on homogenous groups of workers sharing the same working conditions and at a basic level of organisation that allows for action. The research process organised workers' observations of their working conditions and related health problems, (primary workers' experience) into collective experience. This used a questionnaire based on the four 'risk groups'. It was collectively discussed and validated by consensus in the homogeneous group, building also a collective understanding of the complexity of processes and their interrelations. Using this model, the collective analysis is employed to draw a risk map representing the work process, its hazards/ loads and workers' health problems. This is used as a tool for communication with other workers and serves as an instrument to follow changes, positive and negative, at the workplace (Laurell et al., 1992). In a second phase of the investigation, some of the elements detected with the collective questionnaire are verified or quantified using conventional techniques to measure exposure or health outcomes. The final step of a WM study is to determine, again through collective discussion among workers, the priorities for change and the strategies to achieve this, ranging from mobilisation to collective bargaining.

These studies created a widespread consciousness about the importance of work for health that influenced the conception of public health and of health institutions, found in the 1978 Italian Public Health Policy (known as the Sanitary Reform) (Berlinguer, 1979). They also led to a large body of literature on work–health relationships, to changes at the workplace through local action, gave unions and workers greater control over work environment decisions, motivated unions to develop their own occupational health institutions, expanded the areas of local and national collective bargaining agreements to include health issues and motivated changes in labour legislation (Laurell, 1984). The combined effect of these changes contributed to a decline in work-related health problems and work accidents (Berlinguer, 1979).

Latin American participatory occupational health research drew from the Italian WM and from Latin American social medicine, responding to the growing interest in workers' health among both unions and academics in Latin America (Laurell, 1984). Studies have used the WM or a modified version of it called the Collective Questionnaire (CQ) method (Lozano and Noriega, 1984; Rangel and Flores, 1987; Laurell *et al.*, 1992). The CQ method builds on the WM approach but goes further to structure a collective questionnaire to analyse the relationship between work and health. The CQ covers five broad themes: the characteristics of the work process; its hazards/loads; the health damage understood as disorders and diseases it provokes; the existing health protection measures; and those proposed by the workers to protect and promote health. In each of these themes the CQ poses a series of open-ended 'questions or discussion themes' to orient the discussion and facilitate workers' expression of their perceptions, but also allow for some quantification through the proportion of workers exposed to or experiencing health problems

(Frankenhauser and Gardell, 1976). The CQ was also tested against conventional approaches, the comparison of the results of a CQ questionnaire and an individual questionnaire showing a high degree of coincidence (Laurell *et al.*, 1992). The CQ provides qualitative information on the labour process and the risks and health damage of a group of workers, particularly for diseases/disorders that are most problematic for workers or that hinder their ability to work. The CQ establishes simple and complex 'risk health damage' relationships, enables decisions to be made about action and includes discussion on such actions.

The Latin American PR studies generated two types of knowledge that, at least in Latin America, did not exist previously. They elaborated the profile of high levels of work-related ill health and its strong relationship with economic and social conditions that has motivated higher levels of public health attention to this problem. Some studies enabled conclusions on the 'epidemiological profiles' characterising the different types of work processes (Laurell and Marquez, 1983), while others have focused on the impact of technological change and/or changes in labour relations on health. They contributed to bargaining and union-controlled surveillance systems on working conditions and led to the promotion of educational union activities and joint centres on health (Laurell *et al.*, 1992).

Knowledge and change in participatory research

The earlier general discussion and selected examples are used to address the questions:

> Do participatory research methods yield new scientific knowledge in occupational health?
> Have they had an impact on occupational health change?

These two questions are separate but interrelated, as noted by Agris and Schoon (1991) in the fact that research faces the twin issues of rigour and relevance. Once again, it is important to note that this discussion is not a claim for superiority of any method but an examination of the broader choice of approaches to occupational health research. In the discussion that follows it appears that participatory and conventional research approaches can (and sometimes do) usefully interact and that participatory research approaches offer one link between the development of new knowledge and the development of new practice.

The various studies demonstrate that participatory research is a process of scientific inquiry that shifts to varying degrees the involvement in and control of the research process to those who experience the problem investigated. It changes the relationship between the subject (the 'researcher') and object (those under study) of research. In the most radical conception of this approach, the distinction between subject and object is suppressed through the identification of a single 'subject–object', with the 'researcher' as supporter of the process, such as in the Italian WM (Oddone *et al.*, 1969).

This makes the researcher–worker relationship important methodologically *and* in terms of their mutual understanding and interests, control and initiative in the study. Hence, for example, the development of an agreed common 'language' between professionals and workers to mediate the professional expertise of the researcher and the experience of the work (such as the risk groups described earlier). Being a facilitator, consultant, teacher and team member can be challenging for the researcher, and may demand time and additional skills (Mergler, 1987; Greenwood *et al.*, 1992). Participatory research studies may be less easily published in scientific journals as they often concern applied questions and are thus not always regarded as creating new knowledge.

However, from the studies reported here it is evident that participatory research approaches *can and do* add new knowledge, such as in raising the profile of work-related ill health not previously reported or recognised, in outlining the epidemiological profiles characterising different types of work processes, examining the impact of technological change on health, in outlining the cognitive and subjective factors in occupational health exposures and outcomes and in providing a more ecological understanding of work processes and their impact. This latter aspect avoids the single exposure-single disease reductionism and allows for the analysis of multiple outcomes and for the multifactorial relationship between the labour process and health.

Is this knowledge 'scientific'? Frideres (1992) argues that as participatory research does not meet the criteria of being subject to verification by other researchers or evaluated in the light of previous research, and is not the unbiased gathering of information to test a hypothesis, it should not be called scientific. Foot-Whyte (1991) argues however that PR approaches involve the additional rigour of the research being subject to the collective scrutiny and comment of the subjects of the research, often not included in conventional methods. The debate about the scientific nature of PR work is, in our view, a confrontation with theories of epistemology and science that make it difficult to find a simple and adequate answer. It is important, however, to highlight some methodological issues in PR research.

The selection of the study base and of the subjects determines the representativeness of the findings. In many participatory research studies, a census of the organisational unit is selected (for example all workers in a worksite) and few address or report on the issue of non-participation (through unwillingness to participate, lack of access, absenteeism or through domination by certain individuals) and the bias this may lead to in the analysis and interpretation of the results, and in the follow up actions.

Reliability, precision, and the role of random error call for testing of the instruments used to measure exposure and outcomes. This, in fact, becomes even more important in participatory research given the cognitive differences between researchers and workers. Hence, for example, the discussions with workers to elaborate the risk groups in the WM and CQ method, or the collective development of the question-naires and training of unionists in the union-based research.

Systematic misclassification (systematic over- or underreporting of the studied effect in those exposed due to subject or researcher bias) can confound the outcome of studies, including participatory research studies. In PR approaches, it is not appropriate to use conventional control measures, such as 'blind' data collection or external data collectors. Further, methods that use the subjective experience of workers would not view such subjectivity as bias but as substantive information relevant to the research. Such systematic bias becomes problematic, however, if the subjective experience of one group distorts the possibilities of obtaining the subjective experience of another. For example, where groups are homogeneous with respect to the primary occupational health issue being addressed, such as exposure to a work process, but heterogeneous with respect to a dimension that may influ-ence the occupational health problem, such as gender. It is perhaps significant that methods like the WM or CQ provide opportunity for identification of such bias in their inclusion of further investigation by conventional approaches.

The specificity of the information generated to the group studied *does* create problems in the 'external validity' and in the generalis-ability and sustainability of participatory research findings. In many of the PR examples described in this chapter, the restructuring of produc-tion, or work organisation or of production relations made the know-ledge gained through prior PR work unuseful in the new circumstances. Changing external conditions and the practical diffi-culty in sustaining worker mobilisation around occupational health have made specific PR studies unsustainable. The organisational, cultural, cognitive and social context of PR work is thus important information for workers/researchers seeking to understand its relevance in a different workplace or context. It is sometimes the most poorly documented aspect of the research.

These limitations in the scientific 'rigour' of participatory research approaches are, however, counterbalanced by potentials in the 'relevance'. They evidently create a link between the production of knowledge for both the scientific community and for society, establishing new relationships between social groups and the scientific community around knowledge, extending knowledge production beyond the academic domain and the scientific community into the workplace. One of the most significant features of all the PR studies is their link, in a more or less profound way, with changes in production relations and in the work environment. In one process, they combine the identification of risk and the action for its reduction drawing from the perceptions of those exposed to the risk. The assessment of the magnitude of the risk is thus relative to the possibility of acting on it, or what could be termed 'actionable risk'.

In Italy and Sweden, these changes in work environments and in the organisation of occupational health were widespread and substantial. In the more conflictual conditions of Latin America and Africa they have been more localised and vulnerable. In all cases, they have reinforced and supported change through a more direct link between professionals and workers, not simply in the latter using the formers' knowledge, but in a mutual process of generation of knowledge. From our own experience, those involved gain not only the occupational health knowledge obtained in the study, but also a greater level of confidence and capacity to understand, articulate and advance ideas about change in occupational health and in the production process.

The struggles, debates and innovations towards the democratisation of work and work organisation will continue into the twenty-first century. While they are often posed as political or economic questions, this chapter demonstrates that they are also central to occupational health and that occupational health has itself often been a force for democratisation of working life. This presents a challenge to promote research and practice that both explores *and* reflects the importance and the role of participatory approaches in occupational health.

References

Agris, C. and Schoon, D. (1991) 'Participatory action research and action science compared' in W. Foot-Whyte (ed.), *Participatory Action Research*. Newbury Park: Sage.

Alakija, W. (1981) 'Poor visual acuity of taxi drivers as a possible cause of traffic accidents in Bendel state', *Nigeria J. Soc. Occup. Med.*, **31**: 167–70.

Bagnara, S., Misti, R. and Wintersberger, H. (eds) (1985) *Work and Health in the 1980s: Experiences of Direct workers Participation in Occupational Health*. Berlin: Sigma Rainer Bohn Verlag.

Berlinguer, G. (1977) *La Salute nelle Fabbriche*, 7th edn. Bari: De Donato.

Berlinguer, G. (1979) *Una Riforma per la Salute*. Bari: De Donato.

Bioca, M. and Schirripa, P. (1981) *Esperienze di Lotta contra la Nocivita*. Roma: CENSAPI.

Chiaramonte, F. (ed.) (1978) *Sindicato, Ristrutturazione, Organizzazione del Labor.* Roma, Sindicale Italiana.

Fals-Borda, O. (1984) 'Participatory action research in development', *Seeds of Change*, **2**: 18–20.

Fals-Borda, O. (1987) 'The application of participatory action research in Latin America', *Int. Sociology*, **2**(4): 329–47.

Fals-Borda, O. and Rahman, A. (1991) *Action and Knowledge*. New York: Apex.

Fonn, S., Groeneveld, H., De Beer, M. and Becklake, M. (1988) 'Subjective vs objective assessment of exposure to grain dust in relation to lung function in a South African grain mill' in C. Hogstedt and C. Reuterwall (eds), *Progress in Occupational Epidemiology*. Amsterdam: Excerpta Medica.

Foot-Whyte, W. (ed.) (1991) *Participatory Action Research*. Newbury Park: Sage.

Foot-Whyte, W. (1983) 'Worker participation: international and historical perspectives', *Journal of Applied Behavioral Science*, **19**(3): 395–407.

Frankenhauser, M. and Gardell, B. (1976) 'Underload and overload in working life', *Journal of Human Stress*, **35**: 2

Frideres, J. (1992) *Participatory Research Perspectives*, Canada: Captus University Press.

Gardell, B. (1982) 'Worker participation and autonomy: a multilevel approach to democracy at the workplace', *International Journal of Health Services*, **12**: 527–88.

Gardell, B. and Gustavsen, B. (1980) 'Work environment research and social change: current developments in Scandinavia', *J. Occupational Behaviour*, **1**: 3–17.

Garrigou, A., Daniellou, F., Carballeda, G. and Ruaud, S. (1995) 'Activity analysis in participatory design and anlysis of participatory design activity', *Int. J. Ind. Ergonomics*, **15**: 311–27.

Greenwood, D. and Santos, J. (1992) *Industrial Democracy as Process: PAR in the Fago*. Stockholm: Co-operative Group Arbetslivscentrum.

Grisoni, G. and Portelli, H. (1972) *Le Lotte Operaie in Italia*. Milan: Ed. Rizzoli.

Gustavsen, B. (1985) 'Direct workers participation in matters of occupational safety and health: Scandinavan experiences and strategies' in S. Bagnara, R. Misti and H. Wintersberger (eds), *Work and Health in the 1980s. Experiences of Direct Workers' Participation in Occupational Health*. Berlin: Sigma Rainer Bohn Verlag.

Hessel, P.A. and Sluis-Cremer, G.K. (1985) 'The use of lay readers of chest roentgenograms in industrial screening programmes', *J. Occ. Med.*, **27**(1): 43–50.

Johnson, J. and Johansson, G. (eds) (1991) *The Psychosocial Work Environment: Work Organisation, Democratization and Health. Essays in Memory of Bertil Gardell.* New York: Baywood.

Kogi, K. (1991) 'Participatory training for low cost improvements in small enterprises in developing countries' in K. Noro and A. Imada (eds), *Participatory Ergonomics.* London: Taylor & Francis.

Kouabenan, D. (1990) 'Occupational safety and health problems in Cote d'Ivoire', *Int. Labour Review*, **129**(1): 109–19.

Laurell, A.C. (1984) 'Ciencia y experiencia obrera' ('Science and workers experience'), *Cuadernos Politicos*, **41**: 63–83.

Laurell, A.C. and Marquez, M. (1983) *El Desgaste Obrero en Mexico.* Mexico: ERA.

Laurell, A.C. and Noriega, M. (1987) *Trabajo y Salud* in SICARTSA Mexico DF SITUAM and Sindicato Minoer Local 221.

Laurell, A.C., Noriega, M., Martinez, S. and Villegas, J. (1992) 'Participatory research on workers' health', *Social Science and Medicine*, **34**(6): 603–13.

Loewenson, R., Laurell, A.C. and Hogstedt, C. (1994) 'Participatory approaches in occupational health research', *Arbete och Halsa vtenskapligskriftserie*, **38** (Sweden).

Lozano, R. and Noriega, M. (1984) Un mätodo para el estudio de la relacion trabaljo-salud. CICAST, Mexico.

Martin, A. (1992) 'Forward' in A. Sandberg, G. Broms, A. Grip, L. Sundstrom, J. Steen and P. Ullmark (eds) *Technological Change and Co-determination in Sweden.* Philadelphia: Temple University Press.

Mergler, D. (1987) 'Workers participation in occupational health research: theory and practice', *International Journal of Health Services*, **17**(1): 151–67.

Misti, R. and Bagnara, S. (1983) 'La participazione dei lavoratori al controlo e alla prevenzione dei rischi all salute nei luoghi di lavoro', *Medicina dei Laboratori*, **10**(2).

Noro, K. and Imada, A. (eds) (1991) *Participatory Ergonomics.* London: Taylor & Francis.

Noweir, M. (1986) 'Occupational health in developing countries with special reference to Egypt', *American J. Ind. Med.*, **9**: 125–41.

Oddone, I., Marri, G., Gloria, S., Briante, G., Chiatella, H. and Re, A. (1969) *L'Ambiente di Lavoro.* Roma: FIOM-CGIL.

Oleru, U., Kjaduola, G. and Sowho, E. (1990) 'Hearing thresholds in an autoassembly plant prospects for hearing conservation in a Nigerian Factory', *Int. Arch. Occ. Env. Health*, **62**: 199–202.

Ostberg, O., Chapman, L. and Miezio, K. (1991) 'Sailors on the captain's bridge: a chronology of participative policy and practice in Sweden 1945–1990' in K. Noro and A. Imada (1991) (eds), *Participatory Ergonomics.* London: Taylor & Francis.

Raimondi, R. (1985) 'Health and working environment in the Italian industry 1971–1982 workers opinions' in S. Bagnara, R. Misti and H. Wintersberger (eds), *Work and Health in the 1980s. Experiences of Direct Workers' Participation in Occupational Health.* Berlin: Sigma Rainer Bohn Verlag.

Ramirez, R. and Leemans, D. (1985) 'A participative sociotechnical approach to occupational health and safety' in S. Bagnara, R. Misti and H. Wintersberger (eds), *Work and Health in the 1980s. Experiences of Direct Workers' Participation in Occupational Health*. Berlin: Sigma Rainer Bohn Verlag.

Rangel, G. and Flores, A. (1987) *Salud y trabajo secretarial en la UAM Ponencia Encuentro-Seminario sobre Experienciass de investigacion y Vigilanci Epidemiologica cobre*. Mexico: Salud de los Trabajadores.

Tandon, R. (1981) 'Participatory research in the empowerment of people', *Convergence*, **14**(3) 20–9.

Tandon, R. (1988) 'Social transformation and participatory research', *Convergence*, **21**: 5–15.

Wegman, D. and Fine, L. (1990) 'Occupational Health in the 1990s', *Annual Review of Public Health*, **11**: 89–103.

Wintersberger, H. (1985) 'Work and Health' in S. Bagnara, R. Misti and H. Wintersberger (eds), *Work and Health in the 1980s. Experiences of Direct Workers' Participation in Occupational Health*. Berlin: Sigma Rainer Bohn Verlag.

Zwi, A., Fonn, S. and Steinbert, M. (1988) 'Occupational health and safety in South Africa: the perspectives of capital, state and unions', *Social Science and Medicine*, **27**(7): 691–702.

Zimbabwe Congress of Trade Unions (1992) *Report of the Shopfloor Survey on Occupational Health Practices (Part I)*. Mimeo. Harare.

Zimbabwe Congress of Trade Unions (1994) *Report of the Shopfloor Survey on Work Environment Hazards (Part II)*. Mimeo. Harare.

INDEX